INTERMITTENT FASTING MIGHT NOT BE RIGHT FOR WOMEN OVER 50

The Hassle-Free Way to Safely Balance Hormones, Boost Energy, and Lose Weight

EDEN THAYER

Copyright Eden Thayer 2025 - All rights reserved.

The content within this book may not be reproduced, duplicated or transmitted without direct written permission from the author or the publisher.

Under no circumstances will any blame or legal responsibility be held against the publisher, or author, for any damages, reparation, or monetary loss due to the information contained within this book. Either directly or indirectly. You are responsible for your own choices, actions, and results.

Legal Notice:

This book is copyright protected. This book is only for personal use. You cannot amend, distribute, sell, use, quote or paraphrase any part, of the content within this book, without the consent of the author or publisher.

Disclaimer Notice:

Please note the information contained within this document is for educational and entertainment purposes only. All effort has been expended to present accurate, up-to-date, and reliable, complete information. No warranties of any kind are declared or implied. Readers acknowledge that the author is not engaging in the rendering of legal, financial, medical or professional advice. The content within this book has been derived from various sources. Please consult a licensed professional before attempting any techniques outlined in this book.

By reading this document, the reader agrees that under no circumstances is the author responsible for any losses, direct or indirect, which are incurred as a result of the use of the information contained within this document, including, but not limited to errors, omissions, or inaccuracies.

CONTENTS

Introduction	7
1. UNDERSTANDING INTERMITTENT FASTING AND ITS IMPACT ON WOMEN OVER 50	11
The Science Behind Intermittent Fasting	12
How Aging Affects Fasting Outcomes	13
Fasting and Hormonal Balance: What Women Over 50 Need to Know	15
Identifying Risks: Why Intermittent Fasting May Not Be Ideal for Every Woman	17
The Real Talk About Muscle Loss and Fasting: Everything You Need to Know	20
The Not-So-Great News About Fasting and Muscle Loss	22
Your Complete Action Plan for Protecting Muscles While Fasting	23
The Truth About Low Blood Sugar and Fasting: What You Really Need to Know	28
Your Complete Guide to Safer Fasting	31
Let's Talk About Your Bones: Fasting and Bone Health	35
Your Complete Bone Protection Plan While Fasting	38
Fasting and Your Health Conditions: Let's Get Personal	43
The Mental Rollercoaster of Fasting	50
2. HORMONAL HEALTH AND AGING: A COMPREHENSIVE GUIDE	59
Navigating Menopause: Hormonal Shifts Explained	60
The Role of Estrogen and Progesterone in Weight Management	61
How Fasting Interacts with Thyroid Function	65
Beyond Diet: A Holistic Approach	69
Balancing Hormones with Nutrition and Lifestyle	70

3. CUSTOMIZING FASTING APPROACHES FOR INDIVIDUAL NEEDS   73
Creating a Personalized Fasting Schedule   76
Adapting Fasting to Your Lifestyle and Goals   77
Listening to Your Body: When to Adjust or Stop Fasting   79

4. NUTRITION ESSENTIALS FOR FASTING WOMEN OVER 50   83
Crafting Balanced Meals During Eating Windows   85
Recipe Ideas for Fasting-Friendly Meals   87
Supplementation: What You Might Need and Why   91

5. OVERCOMING PSYCHOLOGICAL BARRIERS AND EMOTIONAL EATING   99
Understanding Emotional Eating Triggers   99
Mindful Eating Practices to Support Fasting   101
Building a Positive Mindset with Food   103
Understanding Hunger: Real vs. Psychological   105
Long-term Health Impacts of Intermittent Fasting   107
Fasting Safety: Signs and Symptoms to Monitor   110
Staying Motivated: Tips for Long-term Success   111

6. INTEGRATING EXERCISE WITH FASTING FOR OPTIMAL RESULTS   115
The Truth About Working Out While Fasting: What Women Need to Know   115
The Real Deal About Performance   117
Your Complete Guide to Safer Exercise While Fasting   118
Your Customized Exercise Plans Based on Fasting Style   120
Special Considerations for Different Fitness Levels   121
Nutrition Strategies for Exercise Success   122
Strength Training to Preserve Muscle Mass   124
Cardio and Its Role in a Fasting Routine   126
Recovery and Rest: Essential Components of a Healthy Regimen   128
Why Exercising Fasted May Not Be Ideal for Women   130
Best Practices for Pre-Workout Nutrition   133

7. SOCIAL AND LIFESTYLE CONSIDERATIONS ... 135
   Managing Social Events and Dining Out While Fasting ... 135
   Time Management Tips for Busy Women ... 137
   Fasting and Family: Creating Supportive Environments ... 139
   Adapting Fasting During Travel and Holidays ... 141

8. CASE STUDIES AND SUCCESS STORIES & SOME NOT SO SUCCESSFUL ... 145
   Case Study 1: Success Story: Balancing Hormones and Weight Loss ... 145
   Case Study 2: Overcoming Plateaus: How One Woman Broke Through ... 147
   Case Study 3: Embracing Flexibility: A Journey to Sustainable Health ... 149
   Case Study 4: Susan's Battle with Hormonal Imbalance ... 151
   Case Study 5: Dianne's Struggle with Muscle Loss and Metabolism Slowdown ... 152
   Case Study 6: Maria's Blood Sugar Rollercoaster ... 152
   Community Support: Finding Motivation in Others ... 153

9. EMBRACING A HOLISTIC APPROACH TO HEALTH ... 157
   The Power of Mindfulness and Meditation ... 157
   Stress Management Techniques for Better Health ... 159
   Sleep Optimization: Enhancing Rest and Recovery ... 161
   Building a Holistic Wellness Routine ... 163

10. SELF-COMPASSION AND BODY POSITIVITY ... 167
    Redefining Success: Beyond the Scale ... 169
    Celebrating Small Wins and Progress ... 171
    Developing a Positive Body Image ... 173

11. TOOLS AND RESOURCES FOR CONTINUED SUCCESS ... 177
    Technology at your service ... 177
    Finding Expert Guidance: Coaches and Health Professionals ... 179
    Creating a Personalized Health Journal ... 181
    Building a Support Network for Accountability ... 183

12. SO… SHOULD I INTERMITTENT FAST OR NOT?	187
Finding Your Sweet Spot: Making Fasting Work for You	187
The Big Picture: What We've Learned	188
Making It Sustainable: Your Long-Term Success Plan	190
When Fasting is Unnecessary	194
Your Final Takeaway	199
References	201

INTRODUCTION

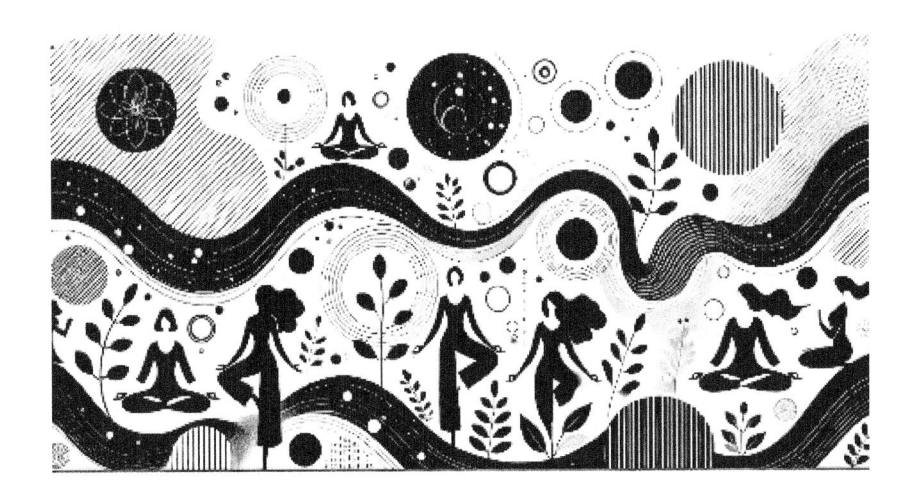

If you're reading this it probably means that you have wondered if intermittent fasting is the right choice for you as a woman over 50. You're not alone. In a world where fasting has gained immense popularity as a weight loss and health improvement strategy, it's natural to feel drawn to its potential benefits. But here's the thing: our bodies change as we age, and what works for a 20-something might not be the best fit for us.

As women, we face unique challenges when it comes to our hormones, especially during perimenopause and menopause. It's a time when our bodies are going through significant shifts, and we need to be extra mindful of how we nourish ourselves. That's why I'm so passionate about helping women like you navigate this journey with confidence and clarity.

Did you know that over 60% of women in their 50s and beyond struggle with hormonal imbalances? It's a staggering number, but it doesn't have to be a life sentence. I've seen firsthand how the right approach to nutrition and self-care can transform lives, and that's what I want to share with you in this book.

While intermittent fasting has its merits, it's not a one-size-fits-all solution. In fact, for some women over 50, it can actually do more harm than good. That's why I've written this book - to help you understand the nuances of fasting, explore alternative methods, and ultimately find what works best for your unique body and lifestyle.

Throughout these pages, we'll dive into the science behind fasting and its impact on women's hormones. We'll explore safe fasting practices, as well as other strategies for balancing hormones, boosting energy, and achieving sustainable weight loss. Each chapter will build upon the last, providing you with a comprehensive roadmap to optimize your health and well-being.

But this book is more than just a guide - it's a conversation. I invite you to reflect on your own experiences and challenges as we navigate this journey together. You'll find practical tips, relatable stories, and a supportive voice that understands what you're going through.

By the end of this book, you'll have a deeper understanding of your body's needs and a toolbox full of strategies to help you thrive. You'll feel empowered to make informed choices about your health, whether that includes intermittent fasting or other approaches tailored to your unique circumstances.

So, are you ready to embark on this transformative journey? To discover how you can safely balance your hormones, reclaim your energy, and achieve your weight loss goals? Then, let's dive in together. Your path to vibrant health starts here.

UNDERSTANDING INTERMITTENT FASTING AND ITS IMPACT ON WOMEN OVER 50

You might recall a time when you could skip a meal here and there without a second thought. Perhaps you even heard a friend rave about a new fasting regimen that promised miraculous results. But as we reach our 50s and beyond, our bodies seem to have a mind of their own. The simple act of not eating for a few hours can feel less like a health strategy and more like a personal challenge. It's not just about willpower; it's about understanding what our bodies need and how they respond to fasting.

For many women, the idea of fasting is alluring. It's natural to hope for a secret weapon against those stubborn pounds that seem to cling a little more each year. But the reality is that as we age, the balance of our hormones shifts, and our metabolism doesn't work quite the same way it used to. This chapter aims to demystify intermittent fasting, exploring what it really means for women over 50. We'll delve into the science, the history, and what you might realistically expect to gain—or lose—from giving it a try.

THE SCIENCE BEHIND INTERMITTENT FASTING

Intermittent fasting is like orchestrating a symphony within your body, where timing is everything. At its core, it involves alternating periods of eating and fasting. During fasting, your body enters a state called autophagy. Think of it as your cells' way of tidying up—removing damaged components to make room for new, healthy ones. This process is crucial for cellular repair and rejuvenation. As we age, our cells' ability to perform these tasks slows down, making autophagy all the more significant.

Fasting also impacts insulin sensitivity and glucose regulation. Insulin, a hormone that helps your body use or store glucose, plays a pivotal role in maintaining energy levels. When you fast, insulin levels drop, which can make your body more efficient at using stored fat for energy. This can be particularly beneficial for those struggling with insulin resistance, a common issue as we grow older.

There's no shortage of methods to choose from when it comes to intermittent fasting. The *16/8 method* is simple: you fast for 16 hours and eat during an 8-hour window. It's popular because it aligns with our natural daily rhythms and doesn't require major lifestyle changes. The *5:2 diet*, on the other hand, involves eating normally for five days a week and significantly reducing calorie intake on the other two. For those who prefer a more structured approach, there's the Eat-Stop-Eat method, which involves a full *24-hour* fast once or twice a week. Each method offers flexibility, allowing you to find what fits best with your life and health goals.

Fasting isn't a new concept. It has deep roots in many religious traditions, where it's seen as a path to spiritual cleansing and discipline. From Ramadan in Islam to Lent in Christianity, fasting has been practiced for centuries. Historically, fasting has also been used for health reasons, dating back to ancient Greece. Today, we continue to explore its benefits, not just for spiritual or cultural reasons, but as a potential tool for managing health.

Many studies highlight the benefits of intermittent fasting. These include weight loss and changes in body composition, such as decreased body fat and increased muscle mass. Improved metabolic markers, like lower blood sugar and cholesterol levels, are also common outcomes. However, while these benefits sound promising, it's crucial to remember that fasting affects everyone differently. What works wonderfully for one person might not work for another, especially when you factor in the unique hormonal landscape of menopause.

Is Fasting Right for You?

Take a moment to think about your current health goals and lifestyle. Are you looking for a method to manage weight more effectively? Or perhaps you're hoping to improve your energy levels and metabolic health? Consider keeping a journal to track your thoughts and experiences if you decide to try intermittent fasting. Note how your body feels, how your mood changes, and any differences in your energy levels. Remember, this book is about helping you find a path that respects your body's needs and celebrates your health at every stage of life.

HOW AGING AFFECTS FASTING OUTCOMES

As we age, our bodies undergo changes that can affect how we respond to fasting. One significant shift is a decrease in basal metabolic rate (BMR), which is the number of calories your body needs to maintain basic physiological functions while at rest. This decrease in BMR means our bodies burn fewer calories than they did in our youth. It's like our internal engine slows down a bit, making it easier for extra calories to turn into stored fat. You may have noticed that you can't eat the same way you did in your thirties without seeing it on the scale. This change can be frustrating, especially when you're trying to lose weight or maintain your current weight.

In addition to a slower metabolism, muscle mass naturally declines as we age, a process known as sarcopenia. Muscle tissue burns more calories than fat tissue, even at rest, so less muscle means fewer calories burned. This shift can lead to changes in body composition, where fat takes up more space, even if your weight remains the same. It's not just about fitting into your favorite jeans; it's about how these shifts can impact your overall health, including your energy levels and physical capabilities. For women over 50, this can mean adjusting how we eat and exercise to support the muscle we have or even gain a little back.

With age comes increased sensitivity to hunger signals. This means that fasting can feel more challenging because the body might respond with stronger hunger pangs. It's not just about willpower; it's a physiological change. You might find that a skipped meal feels more intense than it used to. Recovery after fasting can also take longer. When you're younger, you might bounce back quickly after a fasting period, but as you age, your body might need more time to feel fully replenished. This slower recovery can impact your energy levels, making it harder to stick with a fasting routine.

Hormonal changes also play a significant role in how fasting feels as we age. Cortisol, the stress hormone, can become more unpredictable, often rising during fasting periods. Elevated cortisol levels can lead to increased appetite and cravings, making fasting more challenging. Then there's the duo of leptin and ghrelin—hormones that regulate hunger and fullness. As we age, the balance between these hormones shifts, which can make it harder to recognize when we're truly hungry or full. This imbalance can lead to overeating or feeling unsatisfied after meals, complicating fasting efforts.

For women over 50, fasting poses specific challenges beyond just battling hunger or fatigue. Bone density becomes a concern as estrogen levels drop, increasing the risk of osteoporosis. Fasting, if not managed carefully, might exacerbate this risk if nutritional needs aren't met. Ensuring sufficient intake of calcium and vitamin D becomes crucial, which can be harder to achieve when eating windows are limited. Alongside this, nutrient deficiencies can sneak in if fasting isn't balanced with nutrient-rich meals. It's important to focus on getting a variety of nutrients to support overall health, especially since our bodies might not absorb nutrients as efficiently as they once did.

These physiological shifts mean that fasting for older adults isn't always straightforward. It requires a thoughtful approach that considers individual health needs and lifestyles. It's about finding a balance that supports your health and respects your body's changing needs. When you understand these changes, you can tailor fasting, or any dietary strategy, to better fit your life. It's not about fighting against your body's natural changes but working with them to achieve your health goals.

FASTING AND HORMONAL BALANCE: WHAT WOMEN OVER 50 NEED TO KNOW

As we reach a certain age, our bodies start to communicate in ways they didn't before. Hormones, those tiny chemical messengers, play a starring role in this conversation. For women over 50, especially those navigating menopause, hormones like estrogen and progesterone become central to our health narrative. And when you introduce fasting into the mix, things can get interesting.

Estrogen, often thought of as the "female hormone," does more than we might give it credit for. It influences everything from mood to bone density. During menopause, estrogen levels drop, sometimes dramatically, leading to symptoms like hot flashes, mood swings, and night sweats. Fasting can further affect these levels, sometimes intensifying symptoms or, in some cases, alleviating them. It's a balancing act. Lower estrogen can also impact bone health, increasing the risk of osteoporosis. So, it's not just about managing symptoms but also thinking about long-term health impacts.

Then there's *progesterone*, the often-overlooked companion to estrogen. This hormone helps regulate our cycles and plays a role in maintaining pregnancy. As we age, progesterone levels also decline, which can affect sleep, mood, and even skin health. While fasting, some women may notice changes in how they feel, potentially due to shifts in progesterone levels. It's essential to pay attention to these changes and consider how fasting might be influencing them.

The *thyroid*, a small gland with a big impact, regulates metabolism. It's often underappreciated until something goes awry. Fasting can affect thyroid function, sometimes exacerbating conditions like hypothyroidism, where the gland doesn't produce enough hormones. This can lead to fatigue, weight gain, and even depression. For women over 50 who might already experience these symptoms due to hormonal changes, fasting could amplify these issues. Understanding these interactions is crucial because our goal isn't just to lose weight or feel better temporarily. It's to support our bodies in a way that's sustainable and healthy in the long run.

Balancing hormones isn't just about what we eat—or don't eat. It's also about how we live. A nutrient-rich diet is vital for maintaining hormonal health. Foods rich in omega-3 fatty acids, like salmon and walnuts, can support hormone function. Similarly, leafy greens, whole grains, and lean proteins provide the necessary building blocks for hormones. It's about eating in a way that nourishes our bodies and supports our hormonal health.

Stress management is another key player. *Cortisol*, the stress hormone, can wreak havoc on our bodies, especially when we're stressed. Techniques like meditation, yoga, or even a simple walk can reduce stress levels and help keep cortisol in check. It's not always about finding more time but about using the time we have in ways that support our well-being.

Incorporating these elements into our lives can make a significant difference. It's not about perfection but about making choices that align with our needs and goals. Each of us is unique, and our approach to fasting, diet, and lifestyle should reflect that individuality. Our bodies have supported us through so much; treating them with kindness and respect is the least we can do in return.

IDENTIFYING RISKS: WHY INTERMITTENT FASTING MAY NOT BE IDEAL FOR EVERY WOMAN

Fasting can sometimes feel like a double-edged sword. On one hand, it offers potential benefits that are undeniably appealing. On the other, it comes with risks that we can't ignore, especially as we age.

One of the most pressing concerns is the risk of *hypoglycemia* or low blood sugar. This condition can be particularly worrisome for women who are already managing blood sugar levels due to diabetes or prediabetes. When you fast, your body uses stored glucose for energy, and if your glucose levels dip too low, it can lead to symptoms like dizziness, confusion, and even fainting. It's crucial to understand that while fasting might work wonders for some, it can pose serious health risks for others, especially if those risks aren't properly managed.

Another significant risk is *muscle loss*. As we age, maintaining muscle mass becomes increasingly important, not just for strength but for overall metabolic health. Fasting, particularly if not done carefully, can lead to a decrease in muscle mass. This happens because when your body is deprived of food for extended periods, it might start breaking down muscle tissue to use as energy. This is particularly concerning for older adults, as muscle loss can lead to frailty and decreased mobility over time. This vulnerability highlights the need for a balanced approach to fasting, ensuring that protein intake remains adequate and that strength training is part of your routine.

The impact of fasting on *bone health* during perimenopause and menopause is a crucial consideration, particularly as hormonal shifts make bones more vulnerable to loss. Estrogen plays a key role in maintaining bone density, and as levels decline, the risk of osteoporosis increases. Extended fasting, if not carefully managed, can contribute to inadequate calcium, vitamin D, and protein intake—nutrients essential for bone strength. Additionally, prolonged calorie restriction may increase bone turnover, accelerating loss rather than preservation. It's important to approach fasting with an awareness of these risks, ensuring that nutritional needs are met and that fasting supports, rather than compromises, long-term skeletal health.

Individual health conditions also play a pivotal role in determining whether fasting is appropriate. For instance, managing diabetes while fasting can be a delicate balancing act. It requires careful monitoring of blood sugar levels and possibly adjusting medications. The risk of hypoglycemia is higher, and fasting could complicate diabetes management rather than aid it. Similarly, those with cardiovascular issues must tread carefully. Fasting might affect blood pressure and heart rate, which could exacerbate existing conditions if not monitored closely. It's not just about deciding to fast; it's about understanding how fasting interacts with your health profile.

The *psychological impact* of fasting is another dimension that deserves attention. For many, the idea of restricting food intake can lead to increased anxiety or stress, especially if food has been a source of comfort or control. This heightened focus on when and what to eat can trigger feelings of deprivation or even lead to disordered eating patterns. It's important to recognize these potential mental health implications and address them head-on. Fasting should never feel like a punishment or a source of stress. Instead, it should align with your overall well-being, both mental and physical.

Given these complexities, personalized health assessments become incredibly important. Consulting with healthcare professionals before starting a fasting regimen isn't just a precaution—it's a necessity. They can provide individualized advice based on your medical history, current health status, and personal goals. This tailored approach ensures that fasting if pursued, complements your health rather than jeopardizes it. It's about making informed decisions that prioritize your safety and well-being.

Ultimately, deciding whether intermittent fasting is right for you involves weighing the potential benefits against the risks. It's a deeply personal decision that requires introspection and a willingness to adapt based on what your body needs. A one-size-fits-all approach doesn't work here, and that's perfectly okay. What matters is finding a path that feels right and sustainable for you, whether that includes fasting or not. Your health is a tapestry of choices, and every thread counts.

Let us explore those risks a bit further:

THE REAL TALK ABOUT MUSCLE LOSS AND FASTING: EVERYTHING YOU NEED TO KNOW

Hey there! Let's dive into something that doesn't get enough attention when people talk about fasting – keeping your precious muscles healthy and strong. You know how everyone gets excited about the weight loss benefits of fasting? Well, there's more to the story, especially for those of us who want to maintain our strength and independence as we age.

Why Are We Even Talking About Muscle Loss?

You're excited about starting your fasting journey and seeing all those amazing before-and-after photos online, but nobody mentions that some of that "weight loss" might actually be muscle tissue you'd rather keep. When your body doesn't get food for extended periods, it's like a squirrel looking for nuts in winter – it'll start checking every possible source of energy, including your muscles. This is especially true for those of us over 50, when maintaining muscle becomes about way more than just looking toned in our favorite outfits.

The Science Behind Muscle Loss (In Plain English)

Let's break down what actually happens in your body during fasting. Your body has three piggy banks of energy:

1. The "Quick Cash" Bank: This is your blood sugar and readily available energy
2. The "Savings Account": Your stored glycogen (mainly in liver and muscles)
3. The "Long-term Investment": Your fat tissue

When you fast, your body first breaks into the "Quick Cash" bank. Once that's empty, it moves to the "Savings Account." But here's where it gets tricky – sometimes your body gets a bit too eager and starts breaking down muscle tissue for energy, especially if you're fasting for longer periods. Think of it as your body's panic response: "Help! We need energy! Grab it from wherever you can find it!"

Why Your Muscles Are Worth Their Weight in Gold

Listen, your muscles are doing so much more than helping you open that stubborn jar of pickles (though that's important, too!). Let's talk about why maintaining muscle mass is crucial:

1. **Metabolic Health Superhero**
    - Your muscles are like tiny sugar-processing factories, helping regulate blood sugar and insulin sensitivity
    - The more muscle you have, the more efficient your body becomes at handling carbohydrates
    - This natural blood sugar management system can significantly reduce your risk of type 2 diabetes
    - Muscles actively burn calories even when you're binge-watching your favorite show
2. **Longevity's Best Friend**
    - Studies consistently show that people with more muscle mass tend to live longer
    - Higher muscle mass is associated with better recovery from illness
    - Your muscles help maintain a stronger immune system
    - They provide crucial reserves your body can use during times of stress or illness

3. **Your Independence Insurance Policy**
    - Strong muscles mean better balance (bye-bye, fear of falling!)
    - They help you maintain good posture (hello, confident stance!)
    - Make everyday tasks easier (carrying groceries, playing with grandkids, gardening)
    - Support joint health and reduce the risk of injuries
4. **Bone Density Bodyguard**
    - Muscles pull on bones during movement, stimulating bone strength
    - Weight-bearing exercises that build muscle also increase bone density
    - This combo is your best defense against osteoporosis
    - Better muscle mass means better protection for your joints

THE NOT-SO-GREAT NEWS ABOUT FASTING AND MUSCLE LOSS

Okay, let's talk about what can make muscle loss more likely during fasting. It's like a perfect storm when these factors come together:

Risk Factors for Muscle Loss During Fasting:

1. **Duration of Fasting**
    - Fasting beyond 24 hours significantly increases muscle breakdown risk
    - The longer the fast, the more likely your body is to seek protein from muscles
    - Even shorter fasts can impact muscle if they're not done correctly

2. **Protein Intake Issues**
    - Not getting enough protein during eating windows
    - Poor protein distribution throughout eating periods
    - Low-quality protein sources that don't provide all essential amino acids
3. **Exercise (or Lack Thereof)**
    - No resistance training to signal your body to maintain muscle
    - Overemphasis on cardio without strength training
    - Exercising too intensely while fasted
4. **Hormonal Factors**
    - High cortisol levels from stress
    - Changes in growth hormone production
    - Age-related hormonal changes that already impact muscle maintenance
5. **Overall Nutrition**
    - Insufficient total calorie intake during eating windows
    - Missing key nutrients that support muscle health
    - Poor meal timing relative to exercise

YOUR COMPLETE ACTION PLAN FOR PROTECTING MUSCLES WHILE FASTING

Now for the good news – you absolutely can fast without sacrificing your precious muscle mass. Here's your comprehensive strategy:

1. *Strategic Strength Training*

Your new best friend is resistance training. Here's how to make it work:

Timing Your Workouts:

- Best performed during eating windows when possible
- If training fasted, keep intensity moderate
- Allow adequate recovery time between sessions

Types of Exercise to Include:

- Traditional weight training with dumbbells or machines
- Body weight exercises (pushups, squats, lunges)
- Resistance band workouts
- Pilates or yoga with strength elements
- Functional fitness movements

Weekly Schedule:

- Aim for 2-3 strength sessions per week
- Space them out to allow recovery
- Include all major muscle groups
- Start where you are and progress gradually

2. *Mastering Protein Intake*

Getting enough protein is crucial, but it's not just about how much – it's also about when and what kind.

Daily Protein Goals:

- Aim for 1.0-1.2 grams per kilogram of body weight
- For a 150-pound person, that's about 68-82 grams daily
- Increase slightly if you're very active

Best Protein Sources:

a. Animal-Based Options:
   - Lean meats (chicken, turkey, lean beef)
   - Fish (salmon, tuna, cod)
   - Eggs and egg whites
   - Greek yogurt
   - Cottage cheese
b. Plant-Based Options:
   - Legumes (lentils, beans, chickpeas)
   - Quinoa
   - Tofu and tempeh
   - Nuts and seeds
   - Plant-based protein powders

Timing Your Protein:

- Break your fast with a protein-rich meal
- Space protein intake throughout eating windows
- Consider a protein-rich snack before longer fasting periods

3. *Optimizing Your Fasting Schedule*

Not all fasting protocols are created equal when it comes to muscle preservation.

Recommended Approaches:

- 16:8 method (16 hours fasting, 8 hours eating)
- 14:10 for beginners or those concerned about muscle loss
- 5:2 with adequate protein on both fasting and non-fasting days

- Modified alternate-day fasting with protein-sparing techniques

What to Avoid:

- Extended fasts (>24 hours) without medical supervision
- Aggressive calorie restriction during eating windows
- Combining long fasts with intense exercise

4. *Supplementation Strategies*

While whole foods should be your primary source of nutrients, certain supplements can help:

Consider These Options:

- Essential Amino Acids (EAAs)
- Creatine Monohydrate
- Vitamin D3 (especially if limited sun exposure)
- Magnesium (supports muscle function)
- High-quality protein powder for convenience

5. *Lifestyle Factors for Muscle Preservation*

Don't forget these crucial elements:

Sleep Optimization:

- Aim for 7-9 hours of quality sleep
- Maintain a consistent sleep schedule
- Create a relaxing bedtime routine

Stress Management:

- Practice regular relaxation techniques
- Consider meditation or deep breathing exercises
- Maintain social connections
- Engage in enjoyable activities

Recovery Practices:

- Include rest days between workouts
- Practice gentle movement on rest days
- Use foam rolling or stretching
- Consider massage or other recovery techniques

Warning Signs Your Fasting Might Be Impacting Muscle

Pay attention to these signals:

Physical Signs:

- Decreased strength in regular activities
- Unusual muscle soreness
- Reduced exercise performance
- Slower recovery from workouts
- Visible muscle loss or softening

Energy and Performance Signs:

- Unusual fatigue
- Difficulty completing usual workouts
- Decreased endurance
- Poor concentration

- Mood changes or irritability

When to Adjust Your Approach

Consider modifying your fasting protocol if:

- You're consistently losing strength
- Recovery becomes problematic
- Energy levels remain low
- Sleep quality decreases
- Mood is negatively impacted

The Bottom Line

Remember, fasting can be a powerful tool for health, but it shouldn't come at the cost of your muscle health. By following these comprehensive guidelines and listening to your body, you can maintain and even build muscle while enjoying the benefits of fasting. The key is finding the right balance for your body and lifestyle and being willing to adjust your approach when needed.

THE TRUTH ABOUT LOW BLOOD SUGAR AND FASTING: WHAT YOU REALLY NEED TO KNOW

Let's have a heart-to-heart about something that can make fasting tricky – dealing with low blood sugar, or as medical folks call it, hypoglycemia. You know that shaky, irritable feeling you sometimes get when you've gone too long without eating? That might be your blood sugar talking, and when you're fasting, it's something you definitely want to keep an eye on.

What's Really Happening When Your Blood Sugar Drops?

Think of your blood sugar like your car's fuel gauge. When it starts getting low, things don't run quite as smoothly. In medical terms, we're talking about blood sugar dropping below 70 mg/dL, but you don't need a glucose meter to know something's off. Your body has some pretty clear ways of saying, "Hey, we need some fuel up here!"

Those Tell-Tale Signs Your Blood Sugar's Getting Low:

- That annoying dizzy feeling (like you just got off a merry-go-round)
- Brain fog (when you can't remember where you put your phone... while you're talking on it)
- Suddenly feeling irritable (when even cute puppy videos annoy you)
- Breaking out in a sweat (and no, you haven't been exercising)
- Hands getting shaky (making it hard to text or hold your coffee cup)
- Heart doing a little dance in your chest (palpitations)
- In serious cases, feeling like you might pass out

Why Women Over 50 Need to Be Extra Careful

Here's something nobody really talks about – your body handles blood sugar differently as you age, especially after 50. It's like your body's fuel management system needs a software update, but instead, it's getting a bit glitchy. Here's why:

Age-Related Changes:

- Hormonal shifts (thanks, menopause!) affect how your body processes sugar
- Your insulin sensitivity might not be what it used to be
- Blood sugar regulation becomes less efficient
- Energy needs and metabolism are changing

Extra Risk Factors to Consider:

- Taking certain medications that affect blood sugar
- Having pre-existing conditions like prediabetes
- A history of reactive hypoglycemia (when your blood sugar plays roller coaster)
- Being low in certain nutrients that help regulate blood sugar

The Science of Fasting and Blood Sugar (Without the Complicated Jargon)

Let's break down what happens to your blood sugar during fasting. Think of it like a three-act play:

Act 1: The First 12 Hours

- Your body's using up energy from your last meal
- Blood sugar stays fairly stable
- You're probably feeling pretty good

Act 2: Hours 12-24

- Your liver starts breaking down stored glucose (glycogen)
- It's like breaking into your emergency savings account

- Blood sugar might start getting a bit wobbly

Act 3: Beyond 24 Hours

- Your body switches to burning fat for fuel (hello, ketones!)
- This transition can be bumpy for some people
- Blood sugar regulation becomes more challenging

YOUR COMPLETE GUIDE TO SAFER FASTING

Don't worry – you can absolutely fast safely if you do it right. Here's your comprehensive game plan:

1. *Choose Your Fasting Style Wisely*

Not all fasting methods are created equal. Here are some safer options:

The 12:12 Method

- 12 hours fasting, 12 hours eating
- Perfect for beginners
- Works well with your natural sleep cycle
- Lower risk of blood sugar issues

The 14:10 Approach

- A gentle stretch of the fasting window
- Still allows for good glucose regulation
- Often easier to maintain long-term

Circadian Rhythm Fasting

- Eating with your body's natural clock
- Usually means dinner by sunset
- Helps maintain stable blood sugar levels

2. *Master Blood Sugar Monitoring*

Whether you're using a fancy continuous glucose monitor or regular finger sticks, knowing your numbers can be super helpful:

When to Check:

- Before starting a fast
- If you're feeling symptomatic
- When breaking your fast
- During longer fasting periods

Target Ranges:

- Normal fasting blood sugar: 70-99 mg/dL
- Time to eat: Below 70 mg/dL
- Get help: Below 54 mg/dL

3. *Strategic Meal Planning*

The key to stable blood sugar is what you eat when you're not fasting:

Before Starting a Fast:

- Complex carbs (sweet potatoes, quinoa, oats)
- Healthy fats (avocado, nuts, olive oil)
- Quality protein (helps stabilize blood sugar)

- Fiber-rich foods (they're like time-release energy capsules)

Breaking Your Fast Safely:

- Start with protein and healthy fats
- Add complex carbs gradually
- Avoid sugary foods that can cause a blood sugar spike
- Keep portions moderate

4. *Stay Hydrated (But Do It Right)*

Dehydration can make blood sugar problems worse. Here's how to stay properly hydrated:

During Fasting:

- Plain water (your best friend)
- Herbal teas (unsweetened)
- Mineral water
- Consider electrolytes for longer fasts

What to Avoid:

- Artificial sweeteners (they can mess with blood sugar)
- Caffeine (limit it, as it can affect blood sugar)
- Anything with hidden calories

5. *Create Your Safety Net*

Having a plan for low blood sugar is like having insurance – you hope you won't need it, but you're glad it's there:

Your Emergency Kit:

- Glucose tablets or gel
- Hard candy (for emergencies only)
- Your preferred fast-acting carb
- Phone numbers for emergency contacts

Know When to Stop:

- Severe dizziness
- Confusion
- Extreme weakness
- Heart palpitations
- Feeling like you might faint

Special Considerations for Different Groups

For Those with Diabetes:

- Always consult your healthcare provider first
- More frequent blood sugar monitoring
- Medication adjustments may be necessary
- Shorter fasting windows might be safer

For Those with Prediabetes:

- Start with shorter fasting periods
- Monitor blood sugar more frequently
- Focus on balanced meals when eating
- Pay attention to exercise timing

For Those on Medications:

- Review all medications with your doctor
- Some meds need to be taken with food
- Timing of medications might need adjustment
- Keep a closer watch on blood sugar levels

The Bottom Line on Blood Sugar and Fasting

Fasting can be a powerful tool for health, but it needs to be done with respect for your body's needs, especially when it comes to blood sugar. Remember:

- Listen to your body (it's usually smarter than any fasting app)
- Start slowly and build gradually
- Have safety measures in place
- Don't hesitate to modify or stop if needed
- Work with healthcare providers when needed

The goal isn't to push through at all costs – it's to find a sustainable approach that works for your unique body and situation. Sometimes, that means shorter fasts; sometimes, it means a different eating window; and sometimes, it means deciding that other health approaches might work better for you.

LET'S TALK ABOUT YOUR BONES: FASTING AND BONE HEALTH

Do you know what doesn't get enough attention in the fasting conversation? Your amazing bones! They're literally the framework that keeps you standing tall, and when you're thinking about fasting, you need to know how it might affect these crucial supports. Let's dive into everything you need to know about keeping your bones strong while fasting.

Why Your Bones Matter More Than Ever After 50

First things first – let's talk about what's happening with your bones as you age. Remember when you could jump off the swing set as a kid with no worries? Well, your bones are different now, and here's why:

The Menopause Factor

- Estrogen takes a nosedive (and it's been your bones' best friend all these years)
- Calcium doesn't get absorbed as easily as it used to
- Your bone remodeling process (how bones repair themselves) slows down
- Risk of osteoporosis increases significantly

Think of your bones like a bank account – in your younger years, you were making lots of deposits, but after 50, withdrawals start happening faster than deposits. Now add fasting to the mix, and you've got to be even more strategic about maintaining your bone 'savings.'

How Fasting Could Impact Your Bones

Let's get real about what happens to your bones when you fast. It's a bit like a domino effect:

The Nutrition Challenge

When you're fasting, you might be:

- Missing out on crucial calcium-rich meals
- Not getting enough vitamin D at regular intervals
- Short on other bone-building minerals
- Reducing your overall protein intake (yes, protein matters for bones too!)

The Hormonal Story

Fasting can affect your hormones in ways that matter for bone health:

- Cortisol levels might increase (not great for bone density)
- Growth hormone patterns can change
- Metabolic processes that affect bone maintenance might slow down

The Scientific Scoop on Bones and Fasting

Let's break down what science tells us about fasting and bone health (in plain English, because who needs more complicated stuff?):

What Research Shows:

- Short-term fasting (16 hours or less) usually doesn't cause significant bone problems
- Longer fasts might affect bone metabolism
- The timing of nutrient intake becomes super important
- Exercise during fasting needs special consideration

YOUR COMPLETE BONE PROTECTION PLAN WHILE FASTING

Good news – you can absolutely fast while keeping your bones strong! Here's your comprehensive strategy:

1. *Master Your Mineral Game*

Think of this as your bone-building treasure map:

Calcium Heroes:

- Greek yogurt (perfect for breaking a fast!)
- Sardines (with bones – they're like nature's calcium supplements)
- Dark leafy greens (kale, collards, bok choy)
- Fortified plant milk (if dairy isn't your thing)
- Tofu made with calcium sulfate

Vitamin D Superstars:

- Fatty fish (salmon, mackerel)
- Egg yolks (nature's little vitamin D packets)
- Mushrooms exposed to UV light
- Safe sun exposure (15-20 minutes of morning sun)
- Fortified foods

Other Crucial Players:

- Magnesium-rich foods (nuts, seeds, avocados)
- Vitamin K sources (green leafy vegetables)
- Potassium-packed options (bananas, sweet potatoes)

2. *Time Your Nutrients Right*

When you're not fasting, make every bite count:

Breaking Your Fast:

- Include a calcium-rich food
- Pair it with vitamin D for better absorption
- Add some protein to support bone matrix
- Consider having your largest meal earlier in the day

Before Starting a Fast:

- Eat mineral-rich foods
- Include some healthy fats for vitamin absorption
- Don't skip the protein
- Hydrate well

3. *Exercise Smart*

Your bones need the right kind of movement:

Best Exercises for Bone Health:

- Weight-bearing activities (walking, jogging, dancing)
- Resistance training (starting light and progressing gradually)
- Balance exercises (yoga, tai chi)
- Posture-focused movements

Timing Your Workouts:

- Best done during eating windows when possible
- Keep intensity moderate if exercising while fasted

- Include rest days for recovery
- Listen to your body's signals

4. *Supplementation Strategies*

Sometimes, you need a little extra help:

Consider These (with your doctor's okay):

- Calcium (if you can't get enough from food)
- Vitamin D3 (especially in winter months)
- Vitamin K2 (helps direct calcium to bones)
- Magnesium (supports calcium absorption)

When to Take Them:

- During your eating window
- With food for better absorption
- Spaced out for optimal uptake
- Consistent timing daily

5. *Lifestyle Factors for Better Bone Health*

Don't forget these crucial elements:

Sleep Quality:

- Aim for 7-9 hours nightly
- Keep a consistent sleep schedule
- Create a relaxing bedtime routine
- Use a supportive mattress and pillow

Stress Management:

- Practice relaxation techniques
- Engage in gentle movement
- Maintain social connections
- Find joy in daily activities

Warning Signs to Watch For

Your bones might be trying to tell you something if you notice:

Physical Signs:

- Loss of height (even small amounts matter)
- Changes in posture
- Back pain that wasn't there before
- Bones that seem more sensitive to pressure

Performance Signs:

- Decreased strength in usual activities
- Balance issues
- More frequent falls or near-falls
- Slower recovery from minor impacts

When to Adjust Your Approach

Consider modifying your fasting routine if:

- You have been diagnosed with osteopenia or osteoporosis
- You've had recent fractures
- You're on bone-affecting medications

- You're experiencing unusual bone or joint pain

Special Considerations for Different Groups

For Those with Osteoporosis:

- Shorter fasting windows might be better
- More frequent bone density monitoring
- Extra attention to calcium timing
- Modified exercise programs

For Those on Medications:

- Some medications need to be taken with food
- Others might affect nutrient absorption
- Timing can be crucial for effectiveness
- Always consult your healthcare provider

The Bottom Line on Bones and Fasting

Remember, your bones are playing the long game – they need consistent care and attention. When you're fasting:

- Make your eating windows count nutritionally
- Stay active in bone-healthy ways
- Keep up with preventive care
- Listen to your body's signals

Most importantly, don't let fasting compromise your bone health. If you need to modify your fasting schedule or style to better support your bones, that's not just okay – it's smart!

FASTING AND YOUR HEALTH CONDITIONS: LET'S GET PERSONAL

Let's have an honest conversation about something really important – how fasting plays with different health conditions. Everyone's body is unique. Well, that's especially true when it comes to fasting. What works beautifully for your neighbor might not be the best fit for you, particularly if you're managing specific health conditions.

Fasting with Diabetes: Walking the Tightrope

If you're living with diabetes, you know it's all about balance. Fasting adds another layer to that balancing act, but don't worry – we'll break it down:

The Blood Sugar Balancing Act

Think of managing diabetes while fasting like being a skilled juggler. You're juggling:

- Your normal blood sugar fluctuations
- The effects of fasting
- Your medication timing
- Your activity level
- And sometimes, unexpected curve balls!

What You Need to Know:

- Blood sugar can become less predictable during fasting
- Your medication needs might change
- You'll need to monitor more frequently
- Having a "bail-out" plan is essential

Your Diabetes-Friendly Fasting Strategy

1. **Blood Sugar Monitoring**
    - Check more often than usual (seriously, become best friends with your glucose meter)
    - Keep a detailed log of readings
    - Learn your personal patterns
    - Know your "red flag" numbers
2. **Medication Management**
    - Work with your doctor to adjust the timing
    - Some medications may need dose changes
    - Insulin users need special consideration
    - Keep rescue supplies handy
3. **Meal Planning**
    - Focus on balanced, blood-sugar-friendly meals
    - Time your meals strategically
    - Plan your fasting breaks carefully
    - Keep emergency snacks available

Heart Health and Fasting: Finding Your Rhythm

If you're taking care of your heart, you might be wondering how fasting fits in. Let's get to the heart of the matter (pun intended!):

The Cardiovascular Connection

Your heart doesn't take breaks, so we need to make sure fasting supports rather than stresses it:

What Can Happen:

- Blood pressure might fluctuate
- Heart rate could change
- Electrolyte balance might shift

- Medications might need adjustment

Your Heart-Smart Fasting Plan

1. **Blood Pressure Management**
   - Monitor regularly (especially during fasting periods)
   - Stay hydrated (yes, even when fasting!)
   - Know your warning signs
   - Keep stress levels in check
2. **Medication Timing**
   - Some heart meds need food
   - Others work better on an empty stomach
   - Timing might need adjusting
   - Always consult your cardiologist
3. **Exercise Considerations**
   - Lower intensity during fasts
   - Monitor your heart rate
   - Stay cool and hydrated
   - Listen to your body

Thyroid Tales: Fasting with Thyroid Conditions

Living with a thyroid condition? Your metabolism's already on its own unique journey. Here's how to make fasting work for you:

Understanding the Thyroid-Fasting Connection

Your thyroid is like your body's thermostat, and fasting can affect its settings:

Key Points:

- Metabolism might slow during fasting
- Medication absorption is crucial

- Energy levels need careful monitoring
- Temperature regulation might change

Your Thyroid-Friendly Fasting Strategy

1. **Medication Management**
   - Take thyroid meds on an empty stomach
   - Wait before eating (usually 30-60 minutes)
   - Maintain consistent timing
   - Monitor your symptoms closely
2. **Energy Conservation**
   - Plan activities around energy peaks
   - Rest when needed
   - Don't push too hard
   - Keep warm (your thermostat might be sensitive)

Autoimmune Conditions: Finding Your Balance

Autoimmune conditions add another layer of complexity to fasting. Let's navigate this together:

The Immune System Connection

Your immune system might react differently to fasting:

- Inflammation levels might change
- Energy needs can fluctuate
- Medication timing becomes crucial
- Symptoms might vary

Your Autoimmune-Aware Fasting Plan

1. **Nutrition Strategy**
   - Focus on anti-inflammatory foods

- Time medications carefully
- Monitor symptoms closely
- Have a flare-up plan

2. **Stress Management**
    - Keep stress levels low
    - Practice gentle movement
    - Get adequate rest
    - Stay connected with a support system

Digestive Conditions: Making Peace with Your Gut

Got IBS, acid reflux, or other digestive issues? Here's how to make fasting work for your gut:

Understanding Gut Reactions

Your digestive system might need special consideration:

- Acid production can change
- Motility might shift
- Symptoms could fluctuate
- Medication timing matters

Your Gut-Friendly Fasting Approach

1. **Timing Strategies**
    - Choose fasting windows that match your natural rhythm
    - Break fasts gently
    - Plan for medication timing
    - Listen to your gut (literally!)
2. **Food Choices**
    - Focus on easy-to-digest foods
    - Avoid trigger foods

- Stay hydrated
- Consider probiotics

When Fasting Might Not Be Your Friend

Let's be real – sometimes fasting isn't the best choice. Here's when to think twice:

Absolute No-Go Situations:

- Pregnancy
- Breastfeeding
- Active eating disorders
- Severe illness
- Uncontrolled medical conditions

Proceed with Caution If:

- Recently ill or recovering
- On multiple medications
- Experiencing high stress
- Having active symptoms

Your Personal Health Detective Kit

Here's how to monitor your unique situation:

1. **Keep a Detailed Log**
   - Symptoms
   - Energy levels
   - Medication effects
   - Mood changes
   - Physical responses

2. **Know Your Red Flags**
    - Unusual symptoms
    - Persistent problems
    - Energy crashes
    - Mood changes
    - Sleep disruption
3. **Have a Support System**
    - Healthcare team on speed dial
    - Family and friends who understand
    - Emergency contacts
    - Support groups, if helpful

Making It Work: Your Action Plan

1. **Start Slow**
    - Begin with shorter fasting windows
    - Gradually increase as tolerated
    - Monitor everything
    - Document what works
2. **Be Flexible**
    - Adjust as needed
    - Have backup plans
    - Know when to pause
    - Celebrate small wins
3. **Stay Connected**
    - Regular check-ins with healthcare providers
    - Open communication about challenges
    - Support system awareness
    - Educational resources

The Bottom Line

Remember, having a health condition doesn't automatically rule out fasting – but it does mean you need to be smarter and more strategic about it. Your health journey is unique, and that's okay! The key is finding what works for YOUR body and YOUR conditions.

Most importantly, don't let anyone pressure you into fasting if it doesn't feel right. You're the expert on your body, and sometimes the bravest thing you can do is say, "This isn't right for me right now."

The Mind Game: The Emotional Side of Fasting Nobody Talks About

Let's get real for a minute – fasting isn't just about what happens to your body. It's also a huge mental and emotional journey that can seriously mess with your head sometimes. You know that moment when you're fasting and suddenly every food commercial on TV looks like a masterpiece? Yeah, we need to talk about that and so much more.

THE MENTAL ROLLERCOASTER OF FASTING

Think of fasting like a theme park ride for your emotions. Some days, you're on top of the world, feeling like a willpower warrior, and other days, you're wondering why that stranger's sandwich looks so personally offensive to you. Let's break down what's really going on up there:

The Good Stuff (Yes, There Is Some!)

- That "I've got this!" feeling when you meet your fasting goals

- Mental clarity that sometimes kicks in during a fast
- A sense of accomplishment and control
- Better understanding of your body's signals

The Tricky Bits

- Food thoughts that won't quit (like that pizza place's phone number you suddenly remember from 2003)
- Mood swings that make you question everything
- Social anxiety around food situations
- The emotional rollercoaster of hunger waves

What's Really Going On in Your Head

The Brain-Hunger Connection

Your brain is like that dramatic friend who makes everything into a bigger deal than it needs to be. When you're fasting:

- Your brain might send panic signals ("We're never eating again!")
- Old emotional connections to food surface
- Stress hormones can spike
- Decision-making gets harder

The Emotional Food Web

Let's be honest about our relationship with food:

- It's not just fuel – it's comfort, celebration, and connection
- Fasting can force us to face emotional eating habits
- Social events become more complicated
- Cultural and family food traditions feel challenging

Warning Signs Your Mental Health Might Be Taking a Hit

Red Flags to Watch For:

- Obsessing over food more than usual
- Feeling guilty about eating during your eating window
- Avoiding social situations because of fasting
- Using fasting to punish yourself
- Feeling anxious about breaking your fast
- Getting overly rigid about fasting schedules

Physical Signs of Mental Stress:

- Sleep problems
- Irritability that won't quit
- Anxiety spikes
- Feeling disconnected from your body
- Unusual fatigue
- Mood swings that seem excessive

The Slippery Slope: When Fasting Meets Disordered Eating

This is important, so let's be super clear: fasting should never be a cover for disordered eating patterns.

Watch Out For:

- Using fasting to "make up for" eating
- Extending fasts as punishment
- Competing with others about fasting
- Hiding your eating patterns from others
- Feeling out of control when eating

- Obsessing over fasting apps or trackers

If You Have a History:

- Be extra careful with fasting
- Keep your support team in the loop
- Have clear boundaries and limits
- Know your trigger situations
- Maintain regular check-ins with professionals

Your Mental Health Toolkit for Fasting

1. **Build Your Support System**

Your A-Team Should Include:

- Understanding friends or family
- Healthcare providers who get it
- Maybe a counselor or therapist
- Online or in-person support groups
- Emergency contacts for tough moments

2. **Create Your Coping Strategy Library**

For Those Tough Moments:

- Distraction techniques (that don't involve food!)
- Stress-relief activities you enjoy
- Meditation or breathing exercises
- Physical activities that feel good
- Creative outlets

3. **Develop Your Positive Self-Talk Game**

Replace These Thoughts:

- "I failed at fasting" → "I'm learning what works for me."
- "I can't do this." → "I'm choosing what's best for my body right now."
- "I should be better at this." → "I'm doing the best I can."

4. **Set Up Your Environment for Success**

Make These Changes:

- Clear your space of triggering items
- Create new routines during fasting times
- Plan engaging activities
- Set up a relaxing environment

Practical Strategies for Different Situations

1. **Social Events**

Navigate Them Like a Pro:

- Plan your fasting schedule around important events
- Have ready responses for food offers
- Focus on the social aspect rather than the food
- Know your limits and boundaries

2. **Work Situations**

Office Success Strategies:

- Schedule meetings during your eating window when possible
- Have a plan for office treats and celebrations
- Keep busy during typical snack times
- Prepare responses for food-pushing coworkers

3. **Family Dynamics**

Family Harmony Tips:

- Communicate your needs clearly
- Educate without preaching
- Find ways to participate in food traditions
- Set boundaries with food-pushing relatives

Making Peace with Your Fasting Journey

1. **Practice Self-Compassion**

Remember:

- Everyone's journey is different
- Slip-ups are normal, and human
- Your worth isn't tied to your fasting success
- It's okay to adjust or stop if needed

2. **Stay Flexible**

Your approach should be:

- Adaptable to life changes
- Open to modification
- Free from rigid rules
- Responsive to your needs

3. **Maintain Perspective**

Keep in mind:

- Fasting is a tool, not a lifestyle
- Your mental health matters more than fasting goals
- Perfect fasting doesn't exist
- Your body deserves respect

When to Press Pause or Stop

Consider Taking a Break If:

- Your mental health is suffering
- Anxiety about food is increasing
- Social life is being impacted
- Sleep is disturbed
- Mood is consistently low
- Obsessive thoughts are increasing

Seek Professional Help If:

- Disordered eating patterns emerge
- Depression or anxiety worsen

- You feel out of control
- Fasting is taking over your thoughts
- You're using fasting as punishment

The Bottom Line: Your Mental Health Comes First

Remember this: fasting should enhance your life, not control it. If you're spending more time thinking about fasting than living your life, it's time to reassess. Your mental health is just as important as your physical health – maybe even more so.

Don't be afraid to:

- Adjust your approach
- Take breaks when needed
- Seek professional help
- Change your fasting style
- Stop completely if it's not serving you

Your relationship with yourself is the longest one you'll ever have – treat it with care, respect, and lots of compassion.

HORMONAL HEALTH AND AGING: A COMPREHENSIVE GUIDE

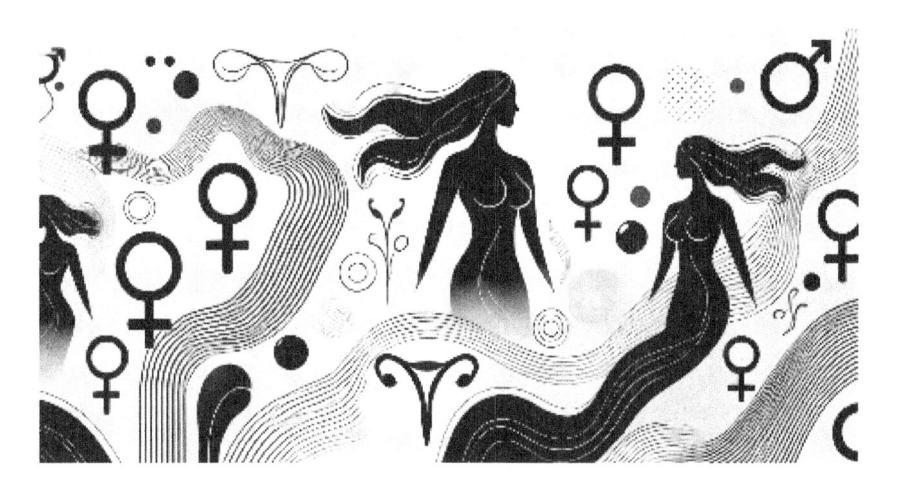

If your body were a finely tuned symphony of gears in a grand clockwork mechanism, with hormones acting as the master cogs that keep everything moving in harmony, as you move through your 50s and beyond, these essential gears may start shifting, slowing down, or speeding up unexpectedly, causing occasional misalignments in the system.

NAVIGATING MENOPAUSE: HORMONAL SHIFTS EXPLAINED

Menopause isn't a sudden event but a gradual process that begins with perimenopause. During this phase, you might notice your hormone levels fluctuating like an unpredictable tide. Your body starts to produce less estrogen and progesterone, leading to changes that can feel bewildering. It's common to experience irregular menstrual cycles, and even some cycles may vanish altogether for a few months, only to return unexpectedly. This period can last several years and often includes symptoms like hot flashes, night sweats, and mood swings. You might find yourself reaching for a fan more often or feeling a bit more irritable than usual. These are all part of the hormonal ebb and flow.

As you transition into menopause, estrogen levels continue to drop, leading to the cessation of menstrual periods. This marks the official onset of menopause. With this decline in estrogen, many women experience a host of symptoms. Hot flashes can become more frequent or intense, and sleep may be elusive, disrupted by night sweats or insomnia. Mood swings can escalate, sometimes leading to periods of depression or anxiety. It's a time when you might feel like you're on an emotional rollercoaster without a clear end in sight. This phase can be challenging, but understanding what's happening hormonally can provide comfort and direction.

After menopause, you enter the postmenopausal stage, where hormonal levels stabilize at lower levels. While some symptoms may lessen, others, like vaginal dryness or changes in libido, can persist. It's important to recognize that these hormonal shifts don't just affect your reproductive system. They have a broader impact on your overall health, including your metabolism. As estrogen falls, your metabolism tends to slow down, which can lead to weight gain. You might notice changes in how your body stores fat, particularly around your abdomen. This isn't just about aesthetics; it's linked to increased risks of metabolic syndrome, hypertension, and diabetes, as highlighted in Source 1.

Understanding these changes is crucial for managing your health effectively. Regular health check-ups become more important than ever. They can help you monitor these shifts and make informed decisions about your health. Hormone Replacement Therapy (HRT) is one option that some women find helpful in alleviating symptoms. However, it's not suitable for everyone and requires careful consideration and consultation with a healthcare provider. It's about finding what balances your unique orchestra and ensures that you feel your best.

Recognizing Your Hormonal Symphony

Take a moment to reflect on your own experiences. Have you noticed changes that align with these hormonal shifts? Consider keeping a journal to track your symptoms and any patterns you observe. This can be a valuable tool when discussing your health with your doctor, helping you make informed choices about potential treatments or lifestyle adjustments. Remember, understanding your hormonal health is not about fixing something that's broken. It's about tuning into your body's needs and responding with compassion and care.

THE ROLE OF ESTROGEN AND PROGESTERONE IN WEIGHT MANAGEMENT

Estrogen is like a finely tuned conductor in the symphony of your body, orchestrating how fat is distributed and stored. When estrogen levels are balanced, they help regulate body fat by influencing where it is stored—whether it ends up as visceral fat, which is deeper and surrounds your organs, or subcutaneous fat, which sits right under your skin. As estrogen levels fluctuate, especially during menopause, you may notice a shift in fat distribution, often settling more around the abdomen. This isn't just a cosmetic concern; visceral fat is linked to higher risks of metabolic diseases. Understanding this can help you make informed decisions about diet and exercise, targeting areas that need more attention for health, not just appearance.

Progesterone, often overshadowed by its more famous partner estrogen, plays a crucial role in managing your hunger and energy use. Think of it as having a calming effect on your brain, subtly regulating your appetite. When progesterone levels dip, as they often do during menopause, you might find your hunger signals getting a bit louder. This hormone also interacts with cortisol, the stress hormone, which can encourage stress-related eating patterns. So, if you find yourself reaching for that extra cookie during stressful times, you're not alone. It's a hormonal dance that affects how you feel and how you eat.

Weight fluctuations during these hormonal shifts can be puzzling. Perhaps you've noticed water retention or bloating, leaving you feeling heavier and more sluggish. These symptoms can be attributed to the hormonal changes you're experiencing. The body responds by holding onto fluids, making your clothes feel tighter, and your energy levels dip. But there are ways to manage these changes without feeling defeated. Recognizing this pattern can help you approach weight management with empathy and understanding, knowing it's not just about willpower but about riding the waves of your body's natural processes.

To manage weight effectively during these times, it helps to focus on hormonal awareness. One practical strategy is incorporating strength training into your routine. This can help counteract muscle loss, which not only boosts your metabolism but also helps reshape your body. Strength training doesn't have to mean heavy lifting; even bodyweight exercises can make a difference. A balanced diet rich in phytoestrogens, which are plant-based compounds that mimic estrogen, can also support weight management. Foods like flaxseeds, soybeans, and berries can be delicious allies in maintaining hormonal balance. They help your body adjust to lower estrogen levels, potentially easing some of the weight-related changes you're experiencing.

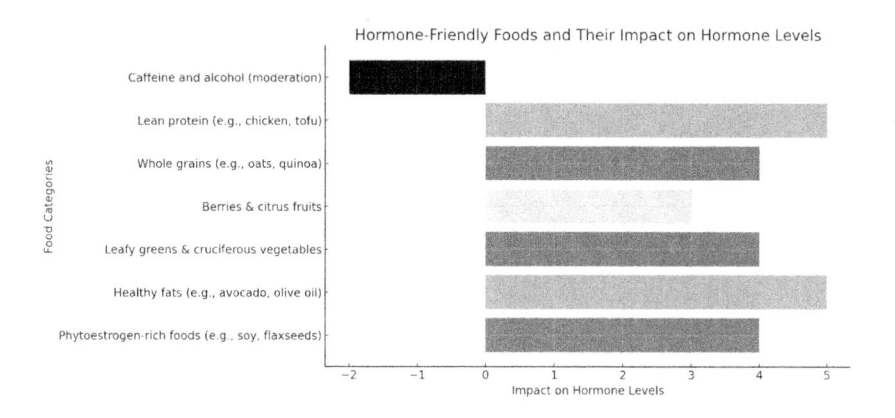

Hormone-Friendly Foods and Their Impact on Hormone Levels

Grey: Represents hormone-friendly foods, which have a positive impact on hormone balance.

Darker shades (dark grey and black): Represent foods that provide more significant benefits, such as healthy fats, phytoestrogens, and lean proteins.

Lighter shades: Indicate foods with moderate positive effects, such as cruciferous vegetables and whole grains.

Comparison of Hormone-Friendly vs Non-Beneficial Foods

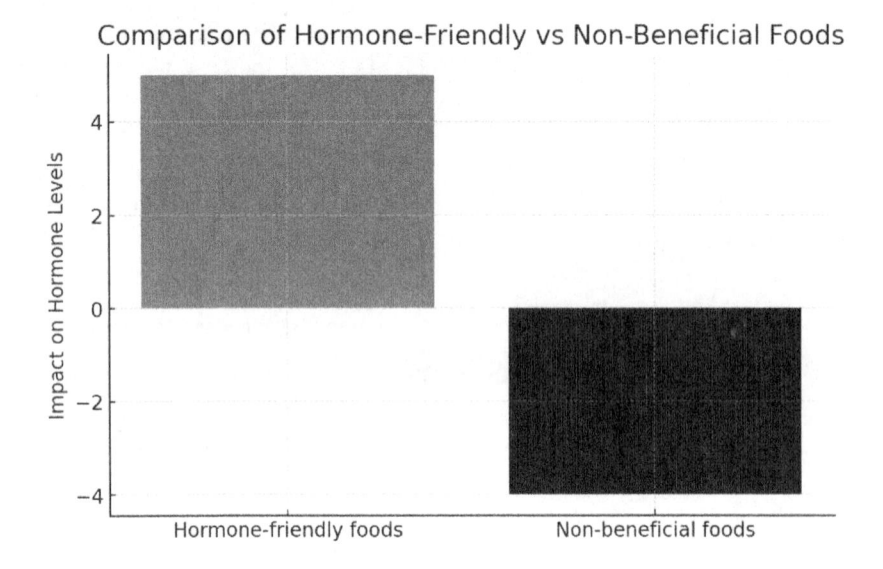

Grey: Represents hormone-friendly foods, which support hormone health.

Black: Represents non-beneficial foods that can disrupt hormonal balance, such as excessive caffeine or alcohol.

Consider setting aside time each week to plan meals that incorporate phytoestrogens and lean proteins. Create a menu that includes dishes like a spinach and tofu stir-fry or a berry and flaxseed smoothie. These meals are not only nourishing but also support your body's hormonal needs. As you plan, pay attention to how different foods make you feel. Does a certain meal leave you feeling energized or sluggish? Use these observations to guide your choices, making adjustments as needed to best support your health.

HOW FASTING INTERACTS WITH THYROID FUNCTION

The thyroid gland, though small, plays a mighty role in our overall health. Nestled in the front of your neck, it functions as a control center for metabolism, regulating how your body uses energy. It produces crucial hormones, mainly T3 (triiodothyronine) and T4 (thyroxine), which are responsible for controlling the speed of your metabolism. Essentially, these hormones determine how fast or slow your body processes calories into energy. If you've ever felt like your energy levels are on a rollercoaster, the thyroid might be behind the scenes. It's involved in everything from how your body burns calories to how your heart beats, making it a key player in keeping your energy levels steady and your metabolism humming along.

Now, when it comes to fasting, things can get a bit tricky for the thyroid. While fasting might offer some benefits, it can also alter the production and balance of thyroid hormones. When the body experiences a calorie deficit, which happens during fasting, it might interpret this as a signal to slow down metabolism to conserve energy. This survival mechanism can lead to a decrease in T3 production, which might explain why some people feel sluggish when they fast. It's a bit like your body putting the brakes on, trying to save fuel for the long haul. This slowdown can be beneficial temporarily, but prolonged periods could potentially disrupt normal thyroid function, especially if your thyroid is already delicate or if you have a history of thyroid issues.

Impact of Fasting on Thyroid Function

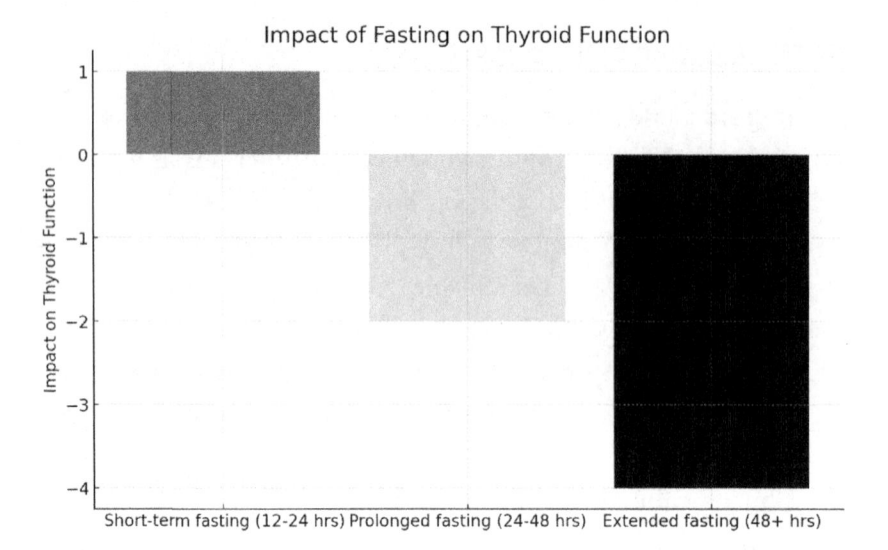

- **Short-term fasting (12-24 hours)**: Generally has a mild positive impact on thyroid function, such as improved insulin sensitivity, but minimal effect on thyroid hormone production.
- **Prolonged fasting (24-48 hours)**: Begins to show a negative impact, with possible decreases in thyroid hormone levels, particularly T3 conversion.
- **Extended fasting (48+ hours)**: Shows a more significant negative impact on thyroid function, as long-term fasting may reduce thyroid hormone production and slow metabolism.

The color gradient represents the varying intensity of the impact, with darker shades indicating a more detrimental effect.

Recognizing the symptoms of thyroid imbalance is crucial, especially if you're exploring fasting.

Key Thyroid Imbalance Symptoms to Watch For During Fasting:

- **Unusual Fatigue & Energy Patterns**: Even after 8+ hours of sleep, you might feel constantly drained. Morning coffee doesn't give the usual kick, and you crash hard by mid-afternoon. Some people describe it as "walking through mud" or feeling like they're always carrying a heavy backpack, even during simple tasks.
- **Hair and Nail Changes**: Your hair might start breaking easily, feel straw-like, or fall out in larger amounts when brushing. Nails often become brittle and develop ridges. These changes happen because thyroid hormones directly affect your body's protein production and nutrient absorption - think of it as your body struggling to maintain its building materials.
- **Skin Transformations**: Beyond just dryness, your skin might become rough, especially on elbows and knees. Some people notice slower healing from cuts or bruises. The skin around your eyes might look puffy, and you could experience increased acne despite good skincare habits.
- **Temperature Sensitivity**: A clear sign is feeling unusually cold when others are comfortable or constantly cold hands and feet. Alternatively, some people experience excessive sweating or heat intolerance. This happens because thyroid hormones regulate your internal thermostat.
- **Weight and Appetite Changes**: You might notice unexplained weight fluctuations despite maintaining your usual eating patterns. During fasting, these changes could

be more pronounced, with either stubborn weight gain or unusual difficulty maintaining weight.
- **Mental Fog**: Beyond physical fatigue, many experience difficulty concentrating, forgetfulness, or slower thinking. It's like trying to read through foggy glasses - everything takes more mental effort than usual.

Nutritional Building Blocks: Feeding Your Thyroid

Think of nutrients as the essential tools your thyroid needs to do its job effectively. Iodine and selenium aren't just fancy words—they're critical players in thyroid hormone production.

Key Thyroid-Loving Nutrients:

- **Iodine**: The foundational building block of thyroid hormones
    - Top sources: Seaweed, fish, dairy, iodized salt
    - Critical for hormone production
    - Balance is key—too little or too much can cause issues
- **Selenium**: The protective guardian of your thyroid
    - Found in: Brazil nuts, fish, eggs, sunflower seeds
    - Helps convert thyroid hormones
    - Acts as an antioxidant, protecting the gland from damage
- **Other Supporting Nutrients**:
    - Zinc: Supports hormone conversion
    - Vitamin D: Crucial for overall thyroid function
    - Iron: Helps in hormone production and metabolism

BEYOND DIET: A HOLISTIC APPROACH

Thyroid health isn't just about what you eat—it's about how you live. Stress, sleep, exercise, and environmental factors all play crucial roles in thyroid function.

Lifestyle Factors That Matter:

- Manage stress through meditation, yoga, or deep breathing
- Prioritize quality sleep
- Engage in regular, moderate exercise
- Minimize exposure to environmental toxins
- Maintain a consistent sleep schedule

The Detective Work: Understanding Thyroid Testing

Think of thyroid blood tests as a comprehensive health report card. It's not just about getting numbers—it's about understanding what those numbers mean for your unique body.

Key Tests to Know:

- **TSH (Thyroid Stimulating Hormone)**: The primary screening test
- **T4 and T3**: Actual thyroid hormones
- **Thyroid Antibodies**: Indicators of autoimmune thyroid conditions

Navigating Test Results:

- Don't just look at numbers—understand their context
- Work with a healthcare provider who listens and explains
- Consider how lifestyle factors might be influencing your results

Lifestyle choices also matter. Stress management can play a significant role in maintaining thyroid health. Chronic stress can lead to elevated cortisol levels, which can interfere with thyroid function. Incorporating stress-reducing activities:

- Manage stress through meditation, yoga, or deep breathing
- Prioritize quality sleep
- Engage in regular, moderate exercise
- Minimize exposure to environmental toxins
- Maintain a consistent sleep schedule

If you're considering fasting, it's wise to approach it with a plan that respects your body's signals and needs. Listening to your body, ensuring you're getting the right nutrients, and keeping an open dialogue with your healthcare provider are steps that can help you maintain thyroid health while exploring fasting.

BALANCING HORMONES WITH NUTRITION AND LIFESTYLE

Navigating the hormonal changes that accompany aging can feel like learning to dance to a new rhythm. Nutrition plays a pivotal role in finding this balance, acting as both a foundation and a support system. *Omega-3 fatty acids* are vital here; they help reduce inflammation in the body, which can minimize the severity of symptoms related to hormonal fluctuations. Foods rich in omega-3s, like salmon, flaxseeds and walnuts, should become staples in your diet. These nutrients not only support brain health but also aid in maintaining a healthy heart, which can be particularly beneficial as we age and our risk for cardiovascular issues increases.

Fiber, too, is a crucial player in this hormonal balancing act. It aids digestion, helps maintain stable blood sugar levels, and can even influence the way your body processes estrogen. Whole grains, fruits, and vegetables are excellent sources of fiber that can support your digestive health and contribute to hormonal equilibrium. By incorporating a variety of these foods into your meals, you not only help keep your digestive system running smoothly but also support your body's ability to regulate hormones more effectively.

Lifestyle changes complement nutritional efforts and are equally important. *Regular physical activity* is a remarkable tool for balancing hormones. It boosts endorphin levels, which can improve mood and mitigate stress. Whether it's a brisk walk, a yoga session, or a dance class, moving your body can help regulate cortisol, the stress hormone, which can often go haywire during menopause. Exercise also promotes better sleep, which is another crucial element in maintaining hormonal health.

Stress management techniques, like yoga and meditation, offer profound benefits for hormonal regulation. These practices encourage mindfulness and relaxation, reducing stress levels that can exacerbate hormonal imbalances. Taking even a few minutes each day to focus on your breath or practice gentle stretching can help tame the chaos that sometimes accompanies hormonal shifts. It's not about achieving perfection in these practices but rather about finding moments of peace that support your overall well-being.

Sleep is another piece of the puzzle that can't be overlooked. Quality sleep is essential for healthy hormone production. During deep sleep, your body releases growth hormones and regulates cortisol levels, helping you wake up refreshed and balanced. Melatonin, the sleep hormone, plays a key role here, guiding your sleep-wake cycle. To improve sleep quality, consider establishing a bedtime routine that signals to your body that it's time to wind down. This could include turning off screens an hour before bed, enjoying a warm bath, or reading a book. Consistency is key, as is creating a sleep environment that is dark, cool, and quiet.

Taking a holistic approach to health management means looking at the big picture and integrating multiple aspects of wellness. It's about combining dietary changes with exercise and mindfulness, creating a lifestyle that supports hormonal health on all fronts. This approach encourages consistency and gradual habit formation, celebrating small victories along the way. By making these changes part of your daily routine, you lay a solid foundation for long-term health and well-being.

Understanding how nutrition, lifestyle, and sleep impact hormone health allows you to take control of your wellness in a new way. These elements create a symphony that, when in harmony, can significantly improve your quality of life. As you continue this exploration, remember that every small change contributes to a healthier, more balanced you. Now, let's look at how we can put these principles into action, creating a personalized plan that fits seamlessly into your life.

CUSTOMIZING FASTING APPROACHES FOR INDIVIDUAL NEEDS

Let's be honest—choosing a fasting method is a lot like dating. You're looking for something that doesn't just look good on paper but actually feels right in your daily life. It's not about finding the trendiest option but discovering something that matches your lifestyle, energy, and personal health goals.

If you were standing in a metaphorical closet of fasting methods, surrounded by different approaches like clothes on hangers, what would you choose? There's the intermittent fasting "little black dress" that seems to work for everyone, the 5:2 diet that looks cute but might feel uncomfortable, and the time-restricted eating that feels like those comfy weekend yoga pants.

At our age, we know one size definitely does not fit all. Our bodies have stories, wisdom, and unique rhythms that can't be ignored. What worked in our 30s might feel like torture now. Some days, you're full of energy and ready to conquer the world. On other days, the thought of restricting anything sounds about as appealing as doing taxes in high heels.

The goal isn't to torture yourself or follow an Instagram-perfect diet plan. It's about finding an approach that makes you feel good, supports your health, and doesn't make you want to throw in the towel after day two. That approach could be gentle and flexible or more structured. The magic is listening to your body and being honest about what works for you.

Think of it like creating a personalized playlist. Some methods will be chart-toppers for you, while others will be total skip-worthy tracks. And that's okay. Your health journey is uniquely yours—no apologies, no guilt, just finding what makes you feel amazing.

Let's explore a few fasting methods that have gained popularity among women in our age group, each with its own flair and function.

Alternate-day fasting...

...is an approach that offers flexibility. On this path, you alternate between days of normal eating and days where you significantly reduce your calorie intake. This method can be appealing if you prefer having some days without any restrictions, allowing you to enjoy social events or family meals without worrying about breaking a fast. It's like giving yourself permission to indulge occasionally, knowing you have a plan in place for the next day. However, this method can present challenges, especially when it comes to managing hunger on fasting days. Ensuring you consume enough nutrients on eating days is crucial to avoid fatigue or nutrient deficiencies.

Time-restricted eating (TRE)...

... is another method, often lauded for its simplicity and alignment with natural circadian rhythms. You eat all your meals within a specific window each day, typically eight to ten hours, and fast for the remaining hours. This method supports the body's natural repair processes during sleep, as fasting can enhance these mechanisms. TRE can be easier to integrate into daily life since it doesn't require drastic dietary changes, and you can adjust your eating window to fit your schedule. However, sticking to a strict eating window might be challenging, especially if your day-to-day life is unpredictable or filled with social commitments that revolve around food.

The 5:2 diet...

...offers moderate calorie restriction. You eat normally for five days of the week and reduce your caloric intake to about 500-600 calories on two non-consecutive days. This method can be attractive if you're looking for a structured yet flexible approach, allowing you to enjoy meals without constant calorie counting. It's like hitting the reset button twice a week. Yet, as with alternate-day fasting, managing hunger and ensuring adequate nutrition on low-calorie days can be difficult. Planning meals that are both satisfying and nutrient-dense is key.

Each method offers potential benefits, from supporting weight management to boosting energy levels and reducing fatigue. These benefits can be particularly appealing as you navigate the changes that come with aging. However, challenges such as managing hunger during fasting periods and ensuring you get enough nutrition can be significant. It's essential to consider your daily schedule, social commitments, and personal comfort with fasting durations when choosing a method.

Assessing Your Fasting Fit

Take a moment to reflect on your lifestyle and health goals. Consider your daily routine, social life, and any health conditions you may have. How do these factors influence your choice of fasting method? Jot down your thoughts in a journal or notebook. This exercise can help you clarify what you need from a fasting regimen and guide you in selecting the method that feels right for you. Remember, the best fasting approach is one that complements your life, not complicates it.

CREATING A PERSONALIZED FASTING SCHEDULE

Creating a fasting schedule that truly fits into your life is a bit like designing a custom wardrobe. You want it to reflect your lifestyle, accommodate your daily routines, and, above all, be comfortable. Start by taking a close look at your current eating habits. Do you find yourself snacking late at night, or is breakfast your favorite meal of the day? Understanding these patterns is crucial in determining your optimal fasting windows. If you're an early riser who enjoys breakfast, perhaps an earlier eating window will suit you best. On the other hand, night owls might prefer a later start. The key is to identify times when fasting feels natural, not forced.

Flexibility is your friend when it comes to sticking with a fasting schedule. Life is unpredictable, and rigid plans often lead to frustration. Consider how your schedule might need to adapt for holidays, family gatherings, or travel. For example, if you have a dinner event, you might adjust your fasting window to start and end later that day. It's about being adaptable and not feeling guilty for making these changes. Embracing this flexibility can help ensure that fasting becomes a sustainable part of your lifestyle rather than a source of stress.

Monitoring your progress is essential to understand if your fasting schedule is working for you. Keeping a journal can be a powerful tool. Note how you feel during and after your fasting periods and any changes in energy levels, mood, or even sleep patterns. This record can reveal patterns or signs that adjustments might be needed. You may be feeling unusually fatigued, which indicates the need to tweak your eating window or the types of foods you consume during meals. Recognizing these signs allows you to make informed decisions, ensuring your fasting plan continues to support your health.

There are numerous resources available to help you on this journey that can ease the process of creating and maintaining a fasting schedule. Digital apps, for instance, can be incredibly helpful. They offer reminders, track fasting intervals, and even provide insights into your progress. Apps like Zero or LifeFasting are designed with flexibility in mind, allowing you to adjust fasting windows as needed. Additionally, sample templates can serve as a starting point, giving you a framework that you can personalize based on your preferences and lifestyle.

Design Your Ideal Fasting Day

Grab a piece of paper or open a note on your phone. Jot down your typical daily schedule, including meal times, work hours, and social activities. Next, sketch out a fasting plan that fits around these elements. Try different configurations until you find one that feels right. This exercise will not only help you visualize your fasting strategy but also make it feel achievable. Remember, the best fasting plan is one that supports your well-being and adapts to the beautiful unpredictability of life.

ADAPTING FASTING TO YOUR LIFESTYLE AND GOALS

When you think about fasting, it's essential to make it work for you, not the other way around. Aligning fasting with your personal goals is crucial because it keeps your efforts meaningful and sustainable. Start by identifying what you want to achieve. Is it weight loss, more energy, or both? Setting clear, achievable objectives will guide your fasting choices and keep you motivated. Weight loss targets should be realistic and tailored to your body's needs, while goals for energy improvement might focus on feeling more vibrant throughout the day. Having these objectives in mind can help you stay on track and measure your progress over time, giving you a sense of accomplishment as you reach each milestone.

Integrating fasting into daily life is about creating a routine that feels natural. Planning meals around fasting windows can help establish consistency. Preparing meals in advance or having a go-to list of fasting-friendly recipes can reduce the stress of last-minute decisions, ensuring you have nutritious options readily available. Balancing fasting with work and family commitments might require some creativity. Perhaps breakfast becomes a shared meal if lunch is skipped, or you enjoy a family dinner within your eating window. The goal is to weave fasting into the fabric of your life, allowing you to maintain your social connections and responsibilities without feeling deprived or isolated.

Social support plays a significant role in fasting success. Involving friends and family can enhance motivation and adherence. Consider creating a support system or joining a fasting group. This community can provide valuable encouragement and accountability. Sharing experiences and recipes with peers can transform fasting from a solitary endeavor into a shared adventure. It can be incredibly rewarding to exchange tips, celebrate successes, and troubleshoot challenges. This network can make fasting feel less like a chore and more like an opportunity to connect and grow with others who understand your journey.

Overcoming lifestyle-related obstacles is part of the process. Social events and busy schedules can present challenges, but they don't have to derail your efforts. Strategies for handling peer pressure to break fasts include politely declining or choosing smaller portions when eating out. You might explain your fasting goals to friends, who will likely respect your choices and may even support you. During holidays or special occasions, maintaining fasting can be tricky. One approach is to adjust your fasting window rather than skipping it entirely. This flexibility allows you to partake in celebrations while staying true to your health goals.

Ultimately, the key is to adapt fasting to suit your life, not the other way around. Remember that fasting is a tool, not a rule. It's there to support your health and enhance your lifestyle, not restrict it. By setting clear goals, integrating fasting into your daily routine, seeking social support, and overcoming obstacles with grace and creativity, you can make fasting a sustainable and rewarding part of your life. It's not about perfection; it's about finding what works for you and embracing the journey toward better health and well-being.

LISTENING TO YOUR BODY: WHEN TO ADJUST OR STOP FASTING

Tuning into your body's signals is crucial when it comes to fasting, especially as we navigate our 50s and beyond. Our bodies have a remarkable way of communicating what they need, but sometimes we overlook these cues in the pursuit of health goals. Recognizing hunger cues and shifts in energy levels can provide valuable insights. If you notice persistent hunger that feels different from the usual pangs, it might be your body's way of telling you it's time for a change. Similarly, if you find your energy levels dipping drastically more than normal, it's worth pausing to consider whether your current fasting routine is serving you well.

There are times when fasting might not be the best fit for your current state. Signs like persistent fatigue or dizziness are red flags that should not be ignored. These symptoms suggest that your body is struggling to cope with the demands of fasting, possibly due to insufficient nutrition or hydration. Emotional distress or heightened anxiety related to fasting can also indicate that it's time to reevaluate. Fasting should never be a source of stress or discomfort. It's important to listen to these signals and consider whether a different approach might be more beneficial.

When it comes to deciding whether to adjust or stop fasting, consulting healthcare professionals can provide valuable guidance. They can help assess whether fasting is impacting your health and suggest modifications that might work better for you. Experimenting with different fasting intervals or methods can also help you find a more comfortable rhythm. Perhaps a shorter fasting window or a different fasting pattern would align better with your body's needs and daily schedule. It's about finding a balance that feels right without compromising your health or well-being.

It's essential to prioritize overall well-being over rigid adherence to fasting rules. Mental health and social connections are just as important as physical health. Fasting should complement your life, not isolate you from it. Make time for activities that nurture your mind and soul, whether it's spending time with loved ones, indulging in a hobby, or simply taking a moment to relax. Integrating self-care practices alongside fasting can create a more holistic approach to health, one that supports you in every aspect of your life.

Valuing your mental health is a crucial aspect of this balanced approach. It's easy to get caught up in the idea that success is measured by how strictly you adhere to a fasting schedule. But true success is about feeling good in your body and mind. Fasting should be a tool that enhances your life, not a regimen that dictates it. If fasting starts to feel like a burden or causes more stress than benefit, it's time to reassess. Remember, there's no one-size-fits-all solution, and it's perfectly okay to try different approaches until you find what works best for you.

As we wrap up this chapter, it's important to remember that your health journey is uniquely your own. Listening to your body and making informed choices about fasting can lead to a more balanced and fulfilling approach to health. As we move forward, we'll explore how nutrition plays a pivotal role in supporting your health and well-being, providing the foundation for a vibrant and energetic life.

NUTRITION ESSENTIALS FOR FASTING WOMEN OVER 50

Have you ever thought about how the food on your plate could be a powerful ally in your quest for hormonal balance and well-being? What we eat can have a profound impact on how we feel, particularly as we navigate the changes that come with age. For women over 50, finding the right nutrients is like discovering the keys to a car that will drive you smoothly through the twists and turns of menopause and beyond. Let's dig into the nutrients that can support your body and help maintain a harmonious balance.

As we age, our bodies often need a little extra support to manage inflammation and stress. *Omega-3 fatty acids* are like tiny warriors fighting inflammation in the body. Found abundantly in fatty fish like salmon and sardines, as well as in walnuts and chia seeds, these healthy fats can help reduce inflammation, which is often a silent culprit behind many health issues. Incorporating omega-3-rich foods into your diet can be a game-changer, particularly if you've noticed joint discomfort or other inflammatory symptoms creeping in.

Magnesium, often dubbed the "relaxation mineral," plays a crucial role in managing stress and improving sleep quality. It's like a gentle balm for the nervous system, helping to calm the mind and relax the muscles. Foods like almonds, spinach, and dark chocolate are excellent sources of magnesium. Including these in your diet can help you manage stress better, which in turn can improve your sleep. And who doesn't appreciate a good night's rest? It's one of the simplest joys that can have a tremendous impact on how we tackle each day.

Vitamin D, the sunshine vitamin, is vital for maintaining strong bones and a stabilized mood. As we age, our ability to produce vitamin D naturally decreases, which can impact bone health and contribute to feelings of fatigue or low mood. Vitamin D can be found in fortified foods such as milk and cereals, as well as fatty fish like salmon. However, sometimes, a little extra help from supplements might be needed, especially during winter months when sunlight exposure is limited. Keeping your vitamin D levels in check can help you maintain your zest for life and protect your bones.

Phytoestrogens are plant-derived compounds found in foods like flaxseeds and soy products that can mimic estrogen in the body. These natural wonders can be particularly beneficial if you're experiencing low estrogen levels, which are common during menopause. Incorporating phytoestrogens into your daily meals can help support hormone regulation. Think of adding a sprinkle of flaxseeds to your morning yogurt or enjoying a stir-fry with tofu. These simple additions can help your body adjust more smoothly to hormonal changes.

Antioxidants are your allies in combating oxidative stress, which can accelerate aging and lead to chronic diseases. Berries like blueberries and strawberries, along with dark leafy greens such as kale and spinach, are packed with antioxidants. By including these foods in your diet, you can help support your body's natural defense system, keeping it robust and resilient. Nuts and seeds also provide antioxidants and are easy to include as snacks. A handful of almonds or walnuts can be a simple yet nutritious way to boost your antioxidant intake.

Incorporating these nutrient-dense foods into your diet doesn't have to be a chore. It can be as easy as adding chia seeds to your smoothies for an omega-3 boost or using turmeric in your cooking to harness its anti-inflammatory properties. These small changes can make a big difference in how you feel day-to-day.

Create Your Nutrient-Rich Meal Plan

Grab a notebook or open a digital note. Write down three meals or snacks you enjoy that could benefit from a nutrient boost. For each, add one of the key nutrients discussed—omega-3s, magnesium, vitamin D, phytoestrogens, or antioxidants. Reflect on how these changes might support your hormonal health and overall well-being.

Remember, nourishing your body is a journey, not a destination. It's about making choices that align with your health goals and enjoying the process of discovering what feels best for you.

CRAFTING BALANCED MEALS DURING EATING WINDOWS

When it comes to eating during your fasting windows, getting the balance right can make a world of difference. Imagine your meals as a well-tuned orchestra, where proteins, healthy fats, and complex carbohydrates play in harmony. Proteins are the strings, providing structure and support, essential for maintaining muscle mass and keeping you satisfied longer. Think of lean meats, beans, or tofu as the backbone of your meals. Healthy fats, like avocados and olive oil, are the brass section, rich and full, offering long-lasting energy and helping your body absorb essential vitamins. Then there are complex carbohydrates, the woodwinds found in whole grains and vegetables, which provide a steady release of energy and keep your blood sugar levels stable. Fiber, our unsung hero, plays the percussion, aiding digestion and ensuring everything moves smoothly. It's found in foods like oats, legumes, and fruits, rounding out your meals and keeping your digestive system happy.

Timing and portion control are equally crucial in this symphony of nutrition. It's about knowing when to strike the right note. Eating within your designated window means getting the most out of every meal. Spread your macronutrients throughout the day to sustain energy levels. Start with a protein-rich breakfast to kick-start your metabolism, followed by a balanced lunch that incorporates all macronutrients. By dinner, you might focus on lighter, easily digestible foods that won't disrupt your sleep. Mindful eating is your conductor's baton, guiding you to savor each bite and helping you recognize when you're full to prevent overeating. Slow down, chew thoroughly, and engage your senses. This not only enhances your eating experience but also aids digestion and helps control portions naturally.

For those of us navigating busy lives, meal planning can feel like an additional chore. Yet, with a few strategies, it can become a time-saver. Batch cooking is a lifesaver—think of it as setting the stage for a week of hassle-free meals. Spend a couple of hours over the weekend preparing staples like grilled chicken, roasted vegetables, or a big pot of soup. Store them in individual portions, ready to grab and go. Quick meals don't have to compromise on nutrition, either. A simple stir-fry with pre-chopped veggies and tofu or a hearty salad with canned beans and a sprinkle of seeds can come together in minutes, keeping you nourished and stress-free.

Maintaining variety in your meals is the spice of life, preventing palate fatigue and keeping mealtime exciting. Embrace the seasons by incorporating fresh, seasonal produce into your dishes. Not only does this enhance flavor and nutritional value, but it also supports local farmers. Rotate your protein sources regularly to keep things interesting—one day, it might be salmon, the next chickpeas, and then perhaps a lean beef stir-fry. By mixing and matching different ingredients, you ensure a wide array of nutrients and keep culinary boredom at bay. Creativity in the kitchen can inspire your taste buds and nourish your body in ways that are both fulfilling and delicious.

RECIPE IDEAS FOR FASTING-FRIENDLY MEALS

Finding meals that fit into your fasting routine can be both exciting and rewarding. The key is to focus on simplicity and nutrition, ensuring that each dish serves a purpose beyond just filling you up.

Overnight Oats: The Ultimate Fast-Breaking Breakfast Solution

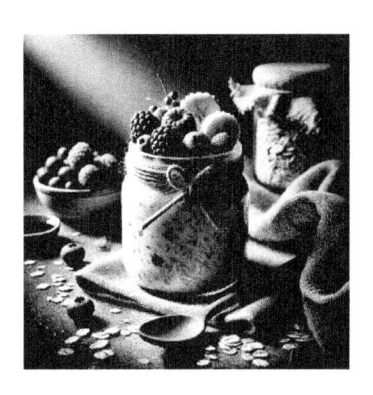

Transform your morning routine with this delightfully simple yet nutritionally powerful meal. Start by combining rolled oats with your choice of milk or yogurt (dairy or plant-based), then add a generous handful of fresh berries. The magic happens overnight in your fridge, where the oats soften and absorb the liquid, creating a creamy, pudding-like consistency that's incredibly satisfying. This breakfast powerhouse not only provides sustained energy through complex carbohydrates but also delivers a significant dose of fiber to support digestive health. The antioxidant-rich berries add natural sweetness while boosting your immune system, making this the perfect way to break your fast with both nutrition and flavor.

Quinoa and Roasted Vegetable Power Bowl: A Symphony of Colors and Nutrients

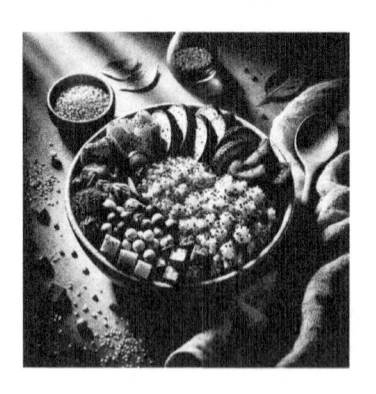

This lunch option celebrates both visual appeal and nutritional density. Begin with a base of protein-rich quinoa, perfectly cooked to fluffy perfection. Layer it with an array of roasted vegetables - sweet bell peppers that provide vitamin C, tender zucchini loaded with potassium, and caramelized sweet potatoes offering beta-carotene. The roasting process brings out the natural sugars in the vegetables, creating deep, complex flavors. Finish with a bright dressing of extra virgin olive oil and fresh lemon juice, which not only enhances the taste but also helps your body absorb the fat-soluble vitamins from the vegetables. This bowl provides steady, sustained energy through its perfect balance of complex carbohydrates and fiber, while the variety of vegetables ensures you're getting a wide spectrum of nutrients.

When it comes to dinner, incorporating meals that support hormonal health is crucial.

Hormone-Supporting Salmon Dinner: A Nutrient-Dense Evening Meal

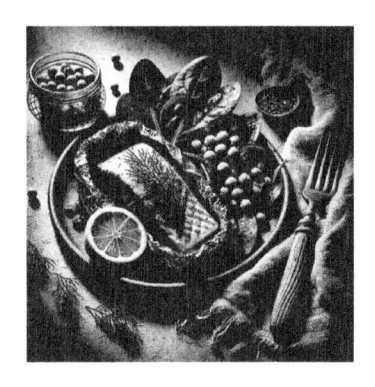

Transform your dinner into a hormone-balancing feast with this thoughtfully crafted salmon dish. The star of the plate is wild-caught salmon, rich in omega-3 fatty acids that support brain health and reduce inflammation. The gentle baking method, wrapped in foil with fresh dill and lemon slices, ensures the fish remains succulent while infusing it with bright, complementary flavors. A side of spinach and chickpea salad adds iron, fiber, and plant-based protein to round out the meal. The combination of leafy greens and legumes provides folate and minerals essential for hormone production, while the healthy fats from the salmon help with nutrient absorption. This dinner not only satisfies your taste buds but also provides crucial nutrients that support your body's natural rhythms.

Plant-Based and Special Diet Options: Inclusive and Flavorful Alternatives

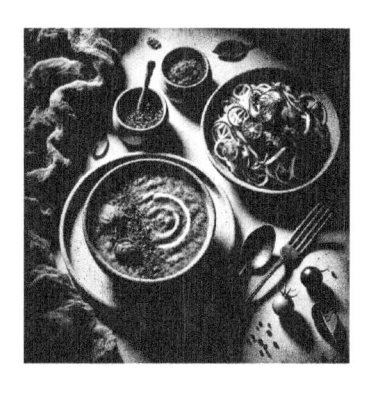

Embrace plant-based eating with a soul-warming bowl of turmeric and ginger lentil soup. This golden bowl of comfort combines protein-rich lentils with anti-inflammatory spices, creating a meal that's both nourishing and healing. The turmeric-ginger combination not only adds depth of flavor but also provides powerful anti-inflammatory compounds that support overall health. For those seeking lighter fare, zucchini noodles with fresh pesto and cherry tomatoes offer a refreshing, gluten-free alternative to traditional pasta dishes. The raw zucchini provides essential enzymes and hydration, while homemade pesto delivers healthy fats and fresh herbs that support detoxification. The addition of sweet cherry tomatoes brings lycopene and a natural umami flavor to the dish.

Customization and Creative Adaptations: Making These Meals Your Own

The beauty of these meal templates lies in their flexibility and adaptability to personal preferences and dietary needs. Don't have quinoa on hand? Brown rice or farro can step in seamlessly, providing similar nutritional benefits with different textures and flavors. Love spicy food? Transform your pesto by adding red pepper flakes or experimenting with different herbs. For the overnight oats, try rotating through different seasonal fruits or adding warming spices like cinnamon and nutmeg. The key is to view these recipes as starting points for your culinary creativity, allowing you to craft meals that not only nourish your body but also bring joy to your eating experience. Remember that sustainable healthy eating comes from finding ways to make nutritious foods exciting and satisfying for your unique palate.

Adjusting recipes to suit your personal tastes is part of the fun. Don't hesitate to swap ingredients based on what you have at home or what you enjoy. If you're not a fan of quinoa, try brown rice or farro in your vegetable bowls. Love a little heat? Add some chili flakes to your pesto. The goal is to create meals that you look forward to and that cater to your dietary needs without compromising on taste. Cooking should be a joy, a chance to experiment and embrace flavors that make you feel good. With these recipes, you're equipped to make choices that align with your health goals while keeping mealtime enjoyable and stress-free.

SUPPLEMENTATION: WHAT YOU MIGHT NEED AND WHY

As we navigate through the complexities of aging, supplementation can become an invaluable ally in ensuring that our nutritional needs are met, especially when fasting. While a balanced diet is the foundation of good health, there are times when dietary supplements might be necessary to fill in the gaps. Multivitamins can be a simple way to cover your bases, ensuring that your body receives a broad spectrum of essential nutrients it might lack. They're like a safety net for those days when your meals might not be as varied as you'd like. Omega-3 supplements, on the other hand, are particularly beneficial if you're not consuming enough fish. These supplements can support heart health and reduce inflammation, offering a convenient way to get those vital fatty acids without having to rely solely on dietary sources.

Women over 50 often face specific nutritional deficiencies that need addressing. Calcium and vitamin D are two such nutrients that are crucial for maintaining bone health. As we age, our bones become more susceptible to thinning, making these nutrients vital for preventing osteoporosis. While you can get calcium from dairy products and vitamin D from sunlight, supplements can ensure consistent intake, especially in winter months or if you're lactose intolerant. B vitamins are another group that supports energy metabolism, helping to convert food into energy more efficiently. They're found in whole grains and leafy greens, but supplementation can be helpful if you're experiencing fatigue or low energy levels.

When selecting supplements, quality is key. It's important to choose reputable brands that offer purity and quality assurance. Reading labels carefully can provide insights into what you're getting—look for third-party testing and certifications that indicate the product has been independently verified. Consulting with healthcare providers is also crucial, as they can offer personalized recommendations based on your health profile. They can help you identify which supplements would be most beneficial for your needs, ensuring that you're not taking anything unnecessary.

Be aware of potential interactions between supplements and medications. Some supplements can affect how medications work, either by enhancing or diminishing their effects. For example, high doses of vitamin K can interfere with blood thinners, while calcium can affect the absorption of certain antibiotics. It's important to check for contraindications with your prescribed medications, and discussing your supplement intake with your healthcare provider can prevent unwanted interactions. Understanding the effects of high-dose supplements is also important, as more isn't always better. Excessive intake of some vitamins and minerals can lead to adverse effects, so it's crucial to stick to recommended dosages.

By being conscious of these factors, you can use supplements to support your health effectively, complementing your fasting routine and ensuring that your body gets everything it needs to function optimally. As you consider which supplements might be right for you, keep in mind that they should enhance, not replace, a healthy diet. They are tools to help you maintain balance and vitality as you continue to explore what works best for your health.

As we conclude this chapter, remember that nutrition and supplementation are just pieces of the puzzle. They work together to support your health, providing the nutrients your body craves while fasting. Embrace this holistic approach, and you'll find yourself feeling more balanced and energized. In the next chapter, we'll delve into overcoming psychological barriers and emotional eating, exploring how your mindset can play a critical role in your health journey.

Multivitamins - Your Comprehensive Daily Insurance Policy When navigating the complexities of fasting and aging, a high-quality multivitamin becomes your nutritional safety net. Think of it as your daily insurance policy, carefully filling potential gaps when meals aren't perfectly balanced. While whole foods should always be your primary source of nutrients, multivitamins offer that extra layer of protection, delivering a carefully calibrated spectrum of essential vitamins and minerals. These supplements become particularly valuable during fasting periods when your eating window is limited, ensuring your body maintains optimal nutrient levels even when your food intake is concentrated into specific times of the day.

Omega-3 Supplements - The Essential Heart and Brain Protector For those who don't regularly include fatty fish in their diet, omega-3 supplements become crucial allies in maintaining health. These powerful supplements provide EPA and DHA, essential fatty acids that support cardiovascular health, reduce systemic inflammation, and contribute to cognitive function. They're particularly valuable during fasting periods when fish consumption might be limited. Look for supplements that provide at least 1000mg of combined EPA and DHA daily, sourced from high-quality fish oil or algae-based alternatives for vegetarians. The anti-inflammatory properties of omega-3s can be especially beneficial during fasting, helping to maintain cellular health and support the body's natural healing processes.

Calcium & Vitamin D - The Dynamic Bone Protection Partnership Women over 50 face unique challenges with bone health, making this supplement duo particularly crucial. While sunlight naturally provides vitamin D and dairy products offer calcium, supplements ensure consistent intake regardless of lifestyle or dietary restrictions. Calcium supplements typically come in doses of 500-600mg, often best absorbed when taken twice daily. Vitamin D, particularly D3 (cholecalciferol), works synergistically with calcium to enhance absorption and support bone mineralization. Aim for 1000-2000 IU of vitamin D3 daily, though needs may vary based on factors like skin tone, sun exposure, and age. This powerful combination becomes even more important during fasting periods when dietary calcium sources might be limited.

B-Complex Vitamins - Your Energy Metabolism Support Team When fatigue becomes a concern, especially during fasting periods, B vitamins can be your metabolic allies. This complex includes eight distinct vitamins (B1, B2, B3, B5, B6, B7, B9, and B12), each playing crucial roles in energy production and nervous system function. While these vitamins occur naturally in whole grains, leafy greens, and animal products, B-complex supplements ensure consistent intake. They're particularly beneficial for vegans and vegetarians who might struggle to get adequate B12 from dietary sources. During fasting, B vitamins help maintain energy levels and support the body's ability to efficiently convert food into usable energy when breaking your fast.

Professional Guidance and Quality Considerations Selecting supplements requires careful consideration of quality and brand reputation. Look for products that have undergone third-party testing and carry certifications from organizations like USP, NSF, or ConsumerLab. These certifications verify that what's on the label matches what's in the bottle. Work closely with healthcare providers to determine optimal dosing based on your individual needs, health status, and any medications you're taking. They can help identify potential interactions - for instance, how vitamin K supplements might affect blood thinners or how the timing of calcium supplements could impact thyroid medication absorption. Regular blood testing can help monitor levels and adjust supplementation as needed.

Safe Supplementation Practices and Integration Understanding proper timing and combinations of supplements maximizes their benefits while minimizing potential interactions. For example, fat-soluble vitamins (A, D, E, K) are best absorbed when taken with meals containing healthy fats. Iron supplements should be taken separately from calcium supplements to ensure optimal absorption. During fasting periods, work with your healthcare provider to determine the best timing for supplements - some may be better taken during your eating window, while others might be suitable during fasting periods. Remember that more isn't always better; excessive intake of certain vitamins and minerals can lead to adverse effects. Always start with recommended dosages and adjust based on professional guidance.

The Holistic Approach to Supplementation Think of supplements as supporting actors in your overall wellness story, working alongside your fasting practice and healthy eating habits. They're designed to complement, not replace, a nutrient-rich diet. This balanced approach creates a strong foundation for addressing the psychological and emotional aspects of health that we'll explore in the next chapter. When your body is properly nourished through both diet and thoughtful supplementation, you're better equipped to handle the mental challenges that might arise during your fasting journey.

Pausing food supplementation can be beneficial as it allows the body to reset and adapt to obtaining essential nutrients from whole foods rather than relying solely on supplements. This break can help prevent potential nutrient imbalances or overconsumption, which may occur when supplements are taken excessively. It also encourages the body's natural absorption mechanisms to function optimally, improving digestion and nutrient utilization. Additionally, taking a break from supplementation can help assess whether the body truly needs certain vitamins or minerals, promoting a more balanced and mindful approach to nutrition. By prioritizing a varied and nutrient-rich diet, individuals can support overall health while reducing dependence on artificial sources of nutrients.

MAKE A DIFFERENCE WITH YOUR REVIEW

Women's solidarity counts!

> *"When you share your knowledge, you help others grow."*
>
> — *UNKNOWN*

If you've been wondering if intermittent fasting is the right choice for you as a woman over 50, you're not alone. I understand how challenging it can be to navigate the changes in our bodies as we age. That's why I wrote this book—to help women like you understand how to balance hormones, boost energy, and lose weight safely, while honoring the unique needs of your body.

Would you help someone just like you embarking on this chapter of her life but unsure where to start?

To reach more women who may be wondering the same thing, I need your help.

Most people choose books based on reviews. So, I'm asking you to take a minute and leave an honest review. It's free, quick, and could be life-changing for someone else. Your review could help:

- One more woman find clarity on what's best for her health
- One more woman regain her energy and balance
- One more woman feel supported and understood during this time of life
- One more woman make informed, confident choices for her well-being

To make a difference, simply scan the QR code below and leave a review:

If you love helping others, you're my kind of person. Thank you from the bottom of my heart for your generosity.

Eden Thayer

OVERCOMING PSYCHOLOGICAL BARRIERS AND EMOTIONAL EATING

Have you ever found yourself reaching for a snack, not out of hunger but because of how you're feeling? Emotional eating is a common experience, one that can sneak up on you during stressful times or when you're feeling down. It's like an old friend who shows up unannounced, offering comfort through food. For many women over 50, this is a familiar pattern, especially as we navigate the changes that come with aging and hormonal shifts. Understanding why we turn to food for comfort is the first step in finding healthier ways to cope.

UNDERSTANDING EMOTIONAL EATING TRIGGERS

Emotional eating often arises from a complex web of psychological and environmental factors. Stress and anxiety, whether from work or family, can drive you to seek solace in food. It can be really overwhelming to navigate a hectic day at work, only to come home and face the demands of family. The stress can flare up, and a quick snack might seem like a small escape. Social pressures during gatherings can also play a role. Perhaps you've felt the subtle nudge to indulge during a dinner party, even when you weren't particularly hungry. It's easy to feel the pull of camaraderie and the expectation to partake in shared meals.

Boredom and a lack of stimulation can be sneaky triggers, too. Those quiet moments when you're alone with your thoughts might lead you to the fridge, seeking something to fill the void. Loneliness or sadness can amplify this pull towards food, turning eating into a source of comfort. You might find yourself reaching for that comforting bowl of pasta or a sweet treat to soothe an emotional ache. These moments can feel isolating, yet they're part of a shared human experience.

Hormonal changes during menopause can further complicate this. Remember how your "need" for certain kinds of food was modified during the menstrual cercle? It can be worse around menopause as the connection between hormone variation and urges is not always clear. As your body undergoes these shifts, you might experience increased cortisol levels, especially during stressful times. This stress hormone can heighten cravings, making you more prone to reach for comfort foods. Meanwhile, fluctuations in serotonin, which affects mood, can also play a role. It's not uncommon to crave carbohydrates or sweets when feeling blue, as these foods can temporarily boost serotonin, offering a fleeting sense of happiness.

The cycle of emotional eating often carries its own emotional weight. After a binge, feelings of shame and regret can wash over you, creating a negative cycle. You might find yourself chastising your lack of control, which only adds to the emotional burden. This guilt can chip away at your self-esteem, making it even harder to break free from the cycle. It's a pattern that can feel relentless, yet it's important to remember that it stems from a natural human desire to soothe discomfort.

To break this cycle, recognizing personal triggers is crucial. Keeping an emotional eating journal can be an invaluable tool. By jotting down what you eat, when, and how you're feeling, you can start to see patterns emerge. This self-reflection can illuminate the connections between your emotions and eating habits, offering insights into your triggers. Practicing self-check-ins before meals can also be helpful. Take a moment to breathe deeply and assess your hunger level. Are you eating because you're physically hungry, or is there an emotional need at play? This pause can be a powerful step in gaining control over emotional eating.

Journaling Your Emotional Eating Patterns

Grab a notebook or open a digital note and begin tracking your eating habits alongside your emotions. Note the date, time, what you ate, and how you were feeling before and after eating. Look for patterns over time and consider how your emotions might be influencing your eating choices. This exercise is not about judgment but about understanding your relationship with food and emotions. As you uncover these patterns, you can start to explore healthier coping mechanisms and make more informed choices about when and what you eat.

MINDFUL EATING PRACTICES TO SUPPORT FASTING

Embracing mindful eating can feel like a revelation, especially when navigating the world of fasting. At its core, mindful eating is about being present and intentional with your food choices. It's more than just eating; it's a full sensory experience. Picture this: you sit down for a meal and really notice the colors, the textures, and the aromas. You take a bite and savor the flavors, paying attention to how the food feels in your mouth. This isn't about rushing through a meal but truly engaging with it. Recognizing true hunger versus habitual eating means you listen to what your body is telling you rather than eating out of routine or boredom.

One way to cultivate mindfulness during meals is by *slowing down*. This may seem simple, but it can be transformative. Start by taking smaller bites and chewing thoroughly. Give yourself permission to enjoy each mouthful.

Before you begin a meal, try engaging in deep breathing. Just a few breaths can help center you, making the transition from a busy day to a peaceful meal. This practice brings awareness to your eating, allowing you to tune into your body's hunger signals. It's a gentle reminder that eating is not just a necessity but a ritual to be cherished.

Mindful eating can significantly enhance your fasting experience. By focusing on the sensory aspects of your meals, you improve your food choices and find greater satisfaction. This approach helps reduce overeating during eating windows as you become attuned to when you're truly full. You might find that you enjoy your meals more, appreciating the flavors and textures in a way you hadn't before. This enjoyment can lead to better digestion and a more positive relationship with food. It's about quality over quantity, making each meal a delightful experience rather than a rushed task.

Developing a routine around mindful eating can be incredibly rewarding. Setting a consistent mealtime schedule helps establish a rhythm, making it easier to incorporate mindfulness into your daily habits. Try to eliminate distractions such as screens during meals. It's tempting to multitask—checking emails or watching TV while eating—but these distractions can detract from the experience. Instead, create a space where meals are an opportunity to disconnect from the busyness of life and reconnect with yourself.

Creating Your Mindful Mealtime Ritual

Consider setting aside a few minutes before each meal to create a mindful mealtime ritual. This could include lighting a candle, playing soft music, or simply taking a few moments to express gratitude for your food. Reflect on the journey your meal took to reach your plate—the farmers who grew it, the journey it took to get to you. This ritual can serve as a bridge between the demands of your day and the nourishment of your body. As you incorporate these practices, notice how they influence your relationship with food and your fasting experience.

BUILDING A POSITIVE MINDSET WITH FOOD

Developing a positive mindset with food is like shifting the lens through which you view nourishment. It's about seeing food as a source of vitality and joy rather than a battleground. When you approach eating with this mindset, it can significantly impact your overall well-being. Think about food as nourishment, providing the essential fuel your body needs to thrive. Instead of punishing yourself with restrictive diets or labeling certain foods as off-limits, embrace the idea that all foods can fit into a balanced lifestyle. This perspective allows you to make choices based on how they make you feel, not on an arbitrary set of rules.

Celebrating the cultural and social aspects of eating can enrich the way you consider food. Meals are more than just sustenance; they're an opportunity to connect with others and with your heritage. Whether it's a family recipe passed down through generations or a new cuisine you're exploring, food has the power to bring people together. By focusing on these aspects, you create a more holistic view of eating that values experiences over restrictions. This can be especially meaningful during gatherings, where sharing a meal becomes a way to strengthen bonds and create memories.

Negative beliefs about food can often stand in the way of developing a healthy mindset about what you eat. One common pitfall is the tendency to label foods as *"good"* or *"bad"* This black-and-white thinking can lead to feelings of guilt or shame when you indulge in something deemed "bad." It's important to recognize that food doesn't have moral value. Instead, consider how different foods make you feel and how they fit into your overall diet. Another harmful belief is associating your self-worth with your dietary choices. You are so much more than the food you eat. Your value isn't determined by whether you had a salad or a slice of cake.

To cultivate *food positivity*, start by practicing gratitude for the nourishment food provides and its journey to your plate. Reflect on the farmers who grew the ingredients, the effort it took to prepare the meal, and the joy it brings. This practice can shift your focus from guilt to appreciation, fostering a healthier mindset. Exploring diverse cuisines can also expand your appreciation for food. By trying new flavors and dishes, you can break free from monotonous eating patterns and find excitement in variety. This exploration can open your palate and your mind, encouraging a more adventurous approach to eating.

Self-compassion and forgiveness are crucial when it comes to overcoming food-related setbacks. It's easy to fall into the trap of self-criticism after overeating or indulging in a treat. However, acknowledging that these moments are part of being human can help you move forward without judgment. Instead of dwelling on what went wrong, consider what you can learn from the experience. Did you eat because you were truly hungry, or was it an emotional response? Reframing setbacks as opportunities for growth allows you to approach them with kindness rather than self-reproach.

Embracing a positive food mindset isn't about perfection but progress.

It's about finding balance and joy in your eating habits and allowing yourself the freedom to enjoy all foods without guilt. By viewing food as a friend rather than a foe, you empower yourself to make choices that nourish both your body and soul. This shift in perspective can lead to a more fulfilling relationship with food, one that celebrates its role in your life and honors your body's needs. As you continue to explore this relationship, remember that every step toward positivity is a victory in itself, bringing you closer to a healthier and more joyful way of living.

UNDERSTANDING HUNGER: REAL VS. PSYCHOLOGICAL

Let's talk about hunger. You know, that gnawing feeling in your stomach that seems to demand your attention, sometimes at the most inconvenient times. But have you ever wondered what's really happening inside your body when you feel hungry? Physiologically, hunger is your body's way of signaling that it needs fuel. This is where hormones like ghrelin and leptin come into play. Ghrelin, often dubbed the "hunger hormone," is produced mainly in the stomach. It sends signals to your brain to indicate hunger, urging you to eat. On the flip side, leptin is produced by your fat cells and works to tell your brain that you're full, helping to regulate energy balance. These hormones work in tandem to maintain a delicate balance between hunger and satiety, ensuring that you consume just enough to meet your body's needs.

However, distinguishing between true hunger and psychological hunger can be tricky. Emotional hunger doesn't stem from physical needs; instead, it often arises from psychological cues. Stress, boredom, and even loneliness can mimic the sensation of hunger, leading you to eat when your body doesn't actually require food. You might recognize this scenario: after a long, stressful day, you're drawn to the fridge not because your stomach is rumbling but because you're seeking comfort. This kind of eating is more about soothing emotions than satisfying physical hunger. The key to unraveling these signals lies in mindfulness and self-awareness. Before reaching for a snack, pause for a moment and ask yourself if you're truly hungry or simply responding to an emotional trigger. This simple question can help you begin to differentiate between the two.

Addressing psychological hunger requires a thoughtful approach. Mindfulness exercises can be incredibly effective. By enhancing your awareness, these practices help you stay present and fully engage with the sensations your body is experiencing. Techniques such as deep breathing or guided meditation can create a moment of pause, allowing you to assess your hunger cues more accurately. Additionally, journaling can serve as a valuable tool for documenting eating triggers and emotions. By keeping a record of what prompts you to eat, you can start to identify patterns and develop strategies to cope with emotional eating urges. This process of reflection can empower you to make more conscious choices about when and what you eat, reducing the grip of psychological hunger.

Creating a hunger management plan tailored to your needs can also be a game-changer. Scheduling regular meal times during your eating windows can help stabilize your hunger signals, making it easier to distinguish between physical and emotional hunger. Consistency trains your body to expect nourishment at certain times, reducing the likelihood of impulsive eating. Additionally, focusing on incorporating filling foods that are high in fiber and protein can keep you satisfied for longer periods.

Think of meals that include whole grains, legumes, lean meats, or plant-based proteins. These foods not only provide sustained energy but also support your overall health and well-being.

Crafting Your Hunger Management Plan

Grab a notebook or open a digital note. Begin by outlining a typical day, noting when you usually eat and how you feel before and after meals. Next, identify any emotional triggers that lead to eating outside of these times. Use this information to develop a personalized hunger management plan. Set specific meal times, choose fiber and protein-rich foods to include, and incorporate mindfulness practices to help you stay aware of your hunger cues. This plan will serve as a guide, helping you navigate the complexities of hunger and making it easier to nourish your body intentionally.

LONG-TERM HEALTH IMPACTS OF INTERMITTENT FASTING

Intermittent fasting has been a hot topic for quite some time, and not just because it's the latest trend. Long-term fasting can offer a suite of health benefits that are particularly compelling for women over 50. One notable advantage is the improvement in insulin sensitivity. As we age, our bodies often become less responsive to insulin, the hormone that helps regulate blood sugar levels. This can lead to higher blood glucose levels and increase the risk of developing type 2 diabetes. Fasting triggers a shift in the way your body processes glucose, potentially lowering blood sugar and enhancing insulin sensitivity. This shift can help stave off diabetes, making fasting a powerful tool in managing long-term health.

But the benefits don't stop with blood sugar. Intermittent fasting can also bolster cardiovascular health, which becomes increasingly important as we grow older. Studies have shown that fasting can lead to lower blood pressure and improved cholesterol levels. Lowering these risk factors can significantly reduce the likelihood of heart disease, which remains a leading cause of health issues in older women. It's like giving your heart a well-deserved break, allowing it to pump more efficiently and effectively. When combined with a balanced diet and regular exercise, fasting can be an integral part of a heart-healthy lifestyle.

On the flip side, there are potential risks associated with long-term fasting that shouldn't be ignored. One such risk is the development of disordered eating patterns. The structure of fasting, with its specific eating windows, might inadvertently encourage an unhealthy focus on food and meal timing. For some, this can spiral into an obsession, leading to anxiety and stress around meals. It's crucial to approach fasting with a mindset focused on health and well-being rather than restriction and deprivation. Listening to your body and maintaining flexibility in your approach can help mitigate these risks.

Mental health is another area where long-term fasting can have mixed impacts. While some people experience improved mental clarity and mood stabilization, others might find that it increases feelings of anxiety or stress. The pressure to adhere to specific eating schedules can be overwhelming, especially if you're juggling multiple responsibilities. It's important to monitor how fasting affects your mental state and to make adjustments as necessary. If fasting starts to feel more like a burden than a benefit, it might be time to re-evaluate your approach.

Current research continues to explore the long-term effects of intermittent fasting, shedding light on its potential anti-inflammatory benefits and impact on aging. Some studies suggest that fasting might help reduce inflammation, a common factor in many chronic diseases. By lowering inflammation, fasting could contribute to a healthier, more resilient body. There's also interest in how fasting might influence the aging process itself. While the jury is still out on whether fasting can extend lifespan, the prospect of aging more healthily is appealing.

Unfortunately, most of the research on intermittent fasting has been conducted on men, with significantly less data available for women—especially women over 50. This is because hormonal fluctuations in women, particularly related to estrogen and progesterone, introduce variables that make studies more complex. Rather than designing research to account for these differences, many studies simply exclude women altogether, leaving a gap in understanding how fasting truly impacts female physiology. What works for men in terms of metabolic benefits and weight loss does not necessarily translate to women, whose bodies respond differently to prolonged fasting, often leading to increased cortisol levels, disrupted sleep, and muscle loss. This lack of research means women are frequently left experimenting with fasting without a clear understanding of whether it is truly beneficial for them or just another trend built on male-centric data.

Given these complexities, medical supervision is crucial for anyone considering long-term fasting. Regular check-ups can help ensure that fasting is not adversely affecting your health. Blood tests can monitor nutrient levels and detect any imbalances early on. Personalized medical advice can provide guidance tailored to your unique health needs, helping you navigate the benefits and risks of fasting. This support can make the difference between a fasting regimen that enhances your life and one that detracts from it.

FASTING SAFETY: SIGNS AND SYMPTOMS TO MONITOR

As you embrace fasting, it's important to keep a close eye on how your body responds. Sometimes, the signals your body sends can be subtle; other times, they're as clear as a sunny day. Persistent dizziness or lightheadedness is one such signal. If you find yourself feeling faint, especially after standing up quickly or during a busy day, it might be your body's way of telling you that it needs a reassessment of your fasting approach. Similarly, if you notice unintentional weight loss that goes beyond your desired goals, it's a red flag. Losing weight too quickly isn't just about clothes fitting differently; it can impact your muscle mass and energy levels, leaving you feeling drained. These symptoms suggest that it might be time to evaluate whether your fasting plan is serving you well or if adjustments are necessary for your health.

Ensuring safety while fasting requires a bit of planning and mindfulness. Staying hydrated is crucial. Sometimes, when you're focused on not eating, it's easy to forget about drinking enough water. But hydration is key to helping your body function smoothly, especially when you're adjusting to a new eating pattern. Keep a water bottle nearby and sip throughout the day. Monitoring your fluid intake can prevent dehydration, which often disguises itself as hunger or fatigue. Additionally, when you start fasting, ease into it gradually. This gentle transition allows your body to adapt without feeling overwhelmed. Start with shorter fasting periods and slowly increase them as your body becomes more accustomed. This approach helps minimize shocks to your system and makes the experience more pleasant.

Listening to your body is a fundamental part of safe fasting. Our bodies have a remarkable way of communicating with us, but we must be willing to listen. If at any point you feel discomfort or distress, it's okay to break your fast. There's no shame in responding to what your body needs. Sometimes, a small snack or a meal is the best choice for your well-being. If you find yourself experiencing adverse effects, it's wise to seek medical advice. A healthcare professional can offer insights and adjustments tailored to your specific needs. Remember, fasting should enhance your life, not complicate it.

For those with pre-existing health conditions, fasting requires extra care and consideration. Each person's health journey is unique, and what's beneficial for one may not be for another. Before starting a fasting regimen, consult with healthcare professionals who understand your medical history. They can help craft a fasting plan that accommodates your conditions and ensures your safety. For instance, if you have diabetes, your fasting approach will differ from someone without this condition. Tailored advice is invaluable in navigating fasting safely and effectively.

As you continue on this path, remember that health is a personal balance, and your body's cues are your guideposts. Being mindful and attentive to these signals allows you to make choices that support your health, leading you to the next chapter.

STAYING MOTIVATED: TIPS FOR LONG-TERM SUCCESS

When it comes to fasting, staying motivated over the long haul can often feel like an uphill battle. That's where intrinsic motivation comes into play. It's that inner drive that comes from genuine interest, not external pressures. Think about what truly motivates you to pursue fasting. Is it a desire to feel more energetic, to embrace a healthier lifestyle, or perhaps to improve your overall well-being? Identifying these personal values and goals is crucial. They serve as your North Star, guiding you through the tougher days when motivation might wane. Keep these reasons close to your heart, and let them be the fuel that keeps you moving forward.

To keep motivation alive, it's important to set small, achievable goals. This isn't about scaling a mountain in one leap but about taking steady, confident steps. Break down your larger goals into bite-sized pieces.

For instance, if your aim is to lose weight, focus on losing a couple of pounds at a time rather than the entire amount. Celebrate each small victory as these achievements build momentum and confidence. Creating a vision board can also be incredibly powerful. Visualizing your goals and the positive outcomes you're striving for can serve as a daily reminder of why you started this journey in the first place. This visual representation can inspire you to keep pushing forward, even on days when the going gets tough.

Community and support are invaluable allies in maintaining motivation. Sharing your experiences with others can uplift and encourage you. Consider joining a fasting support group or an online community where like-minded individuals gather to share stories, challenges, and triumphs. The collective wisdom and camaraderie found in these spaces can provide fresh perspectives and motivate you to stay committed. It's also helpful to have a buddy or two who understand what you're going through. Regularly sharing your progress with friends can keep you accountable and offer emotional support when you need it most. Knowing you're not alone can make all the difference.

Acknowledging and celebrating milestones and achievements is a key component of staying motivated. Reflect on how far you've come and the personal growth you've experienced along the way. Perhaps you're feeling more energetic, or maybe your clothes fit a bit better. These are achievements worth celebrating. Plan non-food-related rewards for reaching your goals. This could be anything from a relaxing spa day to a new book or a fun day out with friends. Celebrating these milestones not only reinforces positive behavior but also makes the journey more enjoyable.

By focusing on intrinsic motivation, setting achievable goals, and embracing community support, you can cultivate a mindset that propels you toward long-term success. Celebrate every step forward, and remember that each day brings new opportunities for progress. As you continue on this path, keep your motivations clear and your support network strong. This foundation will empower you to stay committed and enjoy the process, knowing that you're investing in a healthier, more fulfilling life.

Now, with a solid foundation of motivation and support, we're ready to explore the next chapter, where we delve into integrating exercise with fasting for optimal results, enhancing both physical well-being and the effectiveness of your fasting practice.

INTEGRATING EXERCISE WITH FASTING FOR OPTIMAL RESULTS

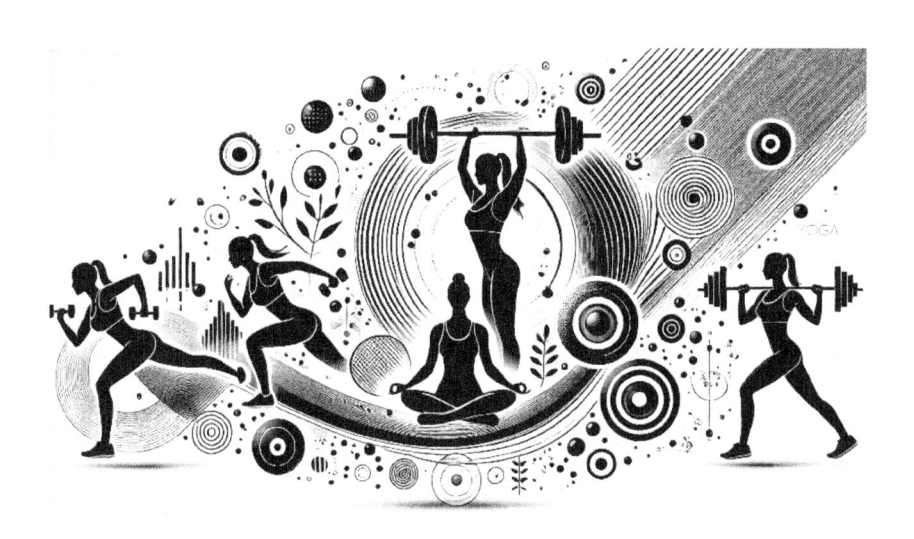

THE TRUTH ABOUT WORKING OUT WHILE FASTING: WHAT WOMEN NEED TO KNOW

Now let's talk about something that might be on your mind – exercising while fasting. You've probably heard all sorts of things, from "never exercise on an empty stomach" to "fasted cardio burns more fat!" But here's the thing: as a woman, your body handles exercise during fasting differently than men's bodies do. Let's dive into what you really need to know.

Why Fasted Exercise Is Different for Women

First things first – let's understand why your body might not be best friends with fasted workouts:

The Hormone Factor

Think of your hormones like a complex orchestra:

- Estrogen and progesterone play leading roles
- Cortisol (stress hormone) gets more reactive when you're fasting
- Your insulin sensitivity is different from men's
- Exercise adds another layer to this hormonal symphony

The Energy Equation

Your body's energy systems are uniquely female:

- Women tend to burn more fat during exercise (even without fasting!)
- You're naturally better at preserving energy (thanks, evolution!)
- Your glucose handling is more sensitive
- Your muscle glycogen gets used differently

THE REAL DEAL ABOUT PERFORMANCE

Let's break down what actually happens when you exercise while fasting:

Strength Training

What Really Happens:

- Power output might decrease
- Recovery can take longer
- Form might suffer if you're low on energy
- Muscle building could be compromised

Cardio Performance

The Truth About Endurance:

- Heart rate might be higher than usual
- Perceived exertion often increases
- Energy availability can be limited
- Recovery needs change

Signs Your Body's Not Happy with Fasted Exercise

Physical Warning Signs:

- Feeling dizzy or lightheaded
- Unusual weakness
- Poor coordination
- Excessive fatigue
- Heart rate that seems off

- Taking longer to recover

Mental Warning Signs:

- Difficulty focusing
- Mood swings during workout
- Feeling overwhelmed easily
- Loss of motivation
- Brain fog that won't quit

YOUR COMPLETE GUIDE TO SAFER EXERCISE WHILE FASTING

1. *Timing Is Everything*

Best Times to Work Out:

- Just before breaking your fast (if doing shorter fasts)
- After your eating window (if you feel energetic)
- During times when you typically feel strongest
- When you have access to food if needed

Times to Avoid:

- Deep into a long, fast
- When you're already feeling depleted
- During very hot weather
- When you're extra stressed

2. *Choose Your Activities Wisely*

Generally Safer Options:

- Walking (especially in nature)
- Gentle Yoga
- Light stretching
- Low-intensity swimming
- Easy cycling

Approach with Caution:

- High-intensity interval training (HIIT)
- Heavy weight lifting
- Long-distance running
- Intense cardio sessions
- Complex movements requiring lots of focus

3. *Master Your Movement Strategy*

Before Your Workout:

- Check-in with your energy levels
- Hydrate well
- Have a backup plan
- Know your limits

During Your Workout:

- Start slowly
- Monitor your heart rate
- Stay extra hydrated
- Listen to your body

- Be ready to modify or stop

After Your Workout:

- Plan your recovery nutrition
- Hydrate even more
- Rest adequately
- Monitor how you feel

YOUR CUSTOMIZED EXERCISE PLANS BASED ON FASTING STYLE

For 16:8 Fasting

Morning Fasters:

- Light movement early in the fast
- Main workout closer to eating window
- Break fast with a protein-rich meal
- Schedule intense workouts after eating

Evening Fasters:

- Exercise during early eating window
- Light movement during fasting period
- Time workouts with energy peaks
- Plan recovery nutrition carefully

For Shorter Fasts (12-14 hours)

- More flexibility with workout timing
- Can handle slightly higher intensity
- Better energy management

- Easier recovery planning

For Longer Fasts (>18 hours)

- Stick to very light movement
- Focus on flexibility and mobility
- Avoid high-intensity work
- Be extra cautious with form

SPECIAL CONSIDERATIONS FOR DIFFERENT FITNESS LEVELS

Beginners

Your Strategy:

- Start with fed exercise
- Gradually experiment with timing
- Keep intensity low
- Focus on form
- Build tolerance slowly

Intermediate Exercisers

Your Approach:

- Mix fasted and fed workouts
- Monitor performance changes
- Adjust based on results
- Keep a detailed log
- Know when to fuel

Advanced Athletes

Your Game Plan:

- Strategic fasting around training
- Careful performance monitoring
- Periodic metabolic testing
- Regular body composition checks
- Professional guidance when needed

NUTRITION STRATEGIES FOR EXERCISE SUCCESS

Pre-Workout (If Breaking Fast)

Timing Options:

- 30-60 minutes before for a small snack
- 2-3 hours before for a larger meal
- Based on workout intensity

Best Choices:

- Easy-to-digest proteins
- Simple carbs, if needed
- Hydration with electrolytes
- Small portions to start

Post-Workout Nutrition

When Breaking Fast:

- Protein-rich foods first
- Add carbs based on workout intensity
- Include electrolytes
- Focus on whole foods

During Continued Fast:

- Know your limits
- Plan your next meal carefully
- Stay extra hydrated
- Monitor recovery

Your Emergency Kit for Fasted Exercise

What to Keep Handy:

- Water bottle with electrolytes
- Small emergency snack
- Blood sugar monitoring tools, if needed
- Phone for emergency contacts
- Medical ID, if relevant

When to Use It:

- Feeling unusually weak
- Experiencing dizziness
- Having trouble focusing
- Feeling uncoordinated
- Just not feeling right

The Bottom Line on Fasted Exercise

Remember these key points:

- Your safety comes first
- Performance might need to take a backseat
- Listen to your body always
- Be willing to adjust your approach
- There's no shame in eating when needed

Most importantly, don't let anyone pressure you into fasted exercise if it doesn't feel right. Your body, your rules! Some women thrive on fasted workouts, while others feel their best exercising after eating. Both approaches are perfectly valid – what matters is finding what works for YOU.

Design Your Fasting-Friendly Workout Plan

Take a moment to jot down your weekly schedule. Identify pockets of time where you can incorporate exercise, considering both your fasting and eating windows. Aim for a mix of low-impact activities like yoga or walking, as well as more vigorous exercises such as strength training. Reflect on how these sessions align with your energy levels and adjust as needed. Your plan should reflect your personal goals and preferences, making exercise a seamless part of your routine. By thoughtfully integrating exercise with fasting, you empower yourself to achieve your health objectives while respecting your body's natural rhythms.

STRENGTH TRAINING TO PRESERVE MUSCLE MASS

Strength training is like giving your body an internal makeover, one that doesn't just enhance your appearance but boosts your health in ways you might not see immediately. As we age, preserving muscle mass becomes a priority, especially during fasting. Muscles play a crucial role in boosting metabolism, which is the rate at which your body burns calories at rest. The more muscle mass you maintain, the higher your resting metabolic rate, which can aid in weight management and overall metabolic health. It's like having a little furnace inside you, burning energy even when you're resting. But the benefits don't stop there. Strength training also improves bone density, a crucial factor for women over 50 who face an increased risk of osteoporosis. By engaging in regular strength exercises, you're not just maintaining muscle but also fortifying your bones, making them stronger and less prone to fractures.

Designing an effective strength training routine doesn't have to be complicated. Focus on compound movements such as squats and deadlifts. These exercises engage multiple muscle groups, making your workouts efficient and comprehensive. Squats, for example, target your legs, core, and even your upper body if you're holding weights. Deadlifts, on the other hand, work the back, glutes, and hamstrings. These movements mimic daily activities, helping you build strength that translates to real-life tasks. If weights seem intimidating, start with bodyweight versions or use resistance bands. These bands provide joint-friendly resistance, making them an excellent choice for those new to strength training or with joint concerns. They're portable and versatile, allowing you to perform a variety of exercises in the comfort of your home.

One of the most powerful exercises is the kettlebell swing. It builds muscle serves also as a cardio exercise. Follow Tracy Reifkind for excellent advice on how to perform correctly, all that you need to know and great workout routines.

Protein is the building block of muscle, and consuming enough of it is vital for muscle preservation, especially when you're fasting.

Timing your protein intake around workouts can maximize its benefits. Consider having a protein-rich snack or meal within an hour after your workout. This timing helps repair muscle fibers and supports muscle growth. Lean meats like chicken or turkey, fish, eggs, and plant-based options like lentils and tofu are excellent sources of high-quality protein. Balancing these with a mix of carbohydrates and healthy fats ensures you provide your body with everything it needs for optimal recovery and energy replenishment.

Progression in strength training is key to continued improvement and avoiding plateaus. Start by gradually adding weight or resistance to your workouts. If you've been lifting the same dumbbells for weeks, try increasing the weight by a few pounds. Listen to your body, and increase resistance only when you feel ready. Incorporating variety in your routine can also keep things interesting and stimulate different muscle groups. Mix up your exercises, add new movements, or change the number of sets and repetitions. This variety prevents your muscles from adapting too quickly, ensuring you continue to see progress and avoid the dreaded plateau.

Strength training during fasting isn't just about lifting weights; it's about empowering yourself to maintain a healthy, active lifestyle. By focusing on building and preserving muscle, you're investing in your health, supporting metabolic function, and fortifying your bones. It's a commitment to yourself and your well-being, one that can pay dividends in energy, strength, and vitality.

CARDIO AND ITS ROLE IN A FASTING ROUTINE

Cardio exercises have long been celebrated for their ability to boost heart health and increase endurance. They rev up your cardiovascular system, making your heart and lungs work harder and more efficiently. But did you know that they can also be a fantastic complement to fasting? Engaging in regular cardiovascular activities can enhance your fitness levels and endurance, which is crucial for maintaining overall health. Cardio helps in burning calories, which supports weight loss and fat reduction, especially when paired with fasting. As your body adapts to this combined approach, you may find yourself feeling lighter and more energetic.

When we talk about cardio for women over 50, it's important to focus on exercises that are effective yet gentle on the body. Walking is a wonderful, low-impact option that you can do anywhere, anytime. It's accessible, requires no special equipment, and offers a chance to enjoy the outdoors. Swimming is another great choice. The water provides resistance, making your muscles work harder while also supporting your joints. If you're looking for something a bit more intense, interval training might be right up your alley. It involves alternating between short bursts of high-intensity activity and periods of rest or low-intensity exercise. This method is efficient for calorie burning and can be tailored to your current fitness level.

Integrating cardio into your fasting schedule requires a bit of planning to ensure you have enough energy without overexerting yourself. Short, moderate-intensity sessions during fasting periods can be beneficial. A brisk walk or a casual bike ride can get your heart pumping without depleting your energy reserves. If you prefer longer or more intense workouts, consider scheduling them during your eating window. This allows you to fuel up before and after the workout, supporting both performance and recovery. The key is to find a balance that works for you, keeping in mind your body's signals and adapting as necessary.

Enjoyment is an often-overlooked factor in sustaining a cardio routine. If you dread your workouts, it becomes a chore rather than a pleasure. Finding activities you genuinely enjoy can transform your fitness routine. Dancing, for instance, is a fun and social way to get your cardio in. Whether it's a solo dance party in your living room or a structured class, moving to music can be incredibly uplifting. Group classes like aqua aerobics offer a social element, making exercise feel less like a task and more like a gathering of friends. The camaraderie and encouragement from others can boost your motivation and make the experience enjoyable.

RECOVERY AND REST: ESSENTIAL COMPONENTS OF A HEALTHY REGIMEN

In the hustle and bustle of everyday life, it's easy to overlook the cornerstone of any successful fitness routine: recovery. We often focus on the workouts themselves, forgetting that rest is where the magic happens. Recovery is not just a break; it's a vital part of the process, allowing your muscles to repair and grow stronger while giving your mind a chance to recharge. Without sufficient rest, the risk of overtraining looms large, potentially leading to injuries that could sideline you for weeks. Overtraining can manifest as chronic fatigue or persistent soreness, signs that your body is crying out for a breather. Integrating rest days into your fitness plan is crucial. These are the days when you let your body heal, adapt, and prepare for the challenges ahead. It's not about being lazy; it's about being smart. A balanced approach ensures that you return to your workouts refreshed and ready to take on new goals.

Optimizing rest and recovery isn't just about taking a day off. It's about actively engaging in practices that enhance your body's ability to heal. Incorporating stretching and flexibility exercises into your routine can work wonders. Stretching helps to reduce muscle tension, improve circulation, and increase your range of motion. It's like giving your muscles a gentle hug, encouraging them to relax and release built-up stress. Foam rolling, also known as self-myofascial release, is another excellent tool. By using a foam roller, you can massage away those pesky knots and tight spots, promoting blood flow and reducing soreness. Both practices can be integrated into your post-workout routine or on rest days, ensuring that your muscles remain supple and ready for action.

Never underestimate the power of sleep in the recovery process. Quality sleep is your body's natural repair shop, where it gets to work on healing and regenerating. During deep sleep, your body releases growth hormones, which play a crucial role in muscle repair and recovery. Establishing a regular sleep schedule can improve the quality of your rest. Going to bed and waking up at the same time each day helps regulate your body's internal clock, making it easier to fall asleep and wake up feeling refreshed. Creating a restful sleep environment is equally important. Your bedroom should be a sanctuary of calm, free from distractions. Consider dimming the lights, keeping the room cool, and using blackout curtains to block out any disruptive light. A comfortable mattress and pillow can also make a significant difference in your sleep quality.

Relaxation techniques are the icing on the cake when it comes to recovery. After a long day or an intense workout, practicing mindfulness or meditation can help calm your mind and body. These practices encourage you to focus on the present moment, reducing stress and anxiety. Even a few minutes of deep breathing can lower your heart rate and promote relaxation. Engaging in restorative yoga is another great option. This gentle form of yoga focuses on holding poses for extended periods, allowing your body to release tension and stress. It's a perfect way to wind down after a busy day, leaving you feeling centered and at peace.

Recovery and rest are essential, not just as part of a fitness routine but as integral components of a healthy lifestyle. By prioritizing rest, you're not only caring for your body but also nurturing your mind. In the next chapter, we'll explore how social and lifestyle considerations can further support your health goals, ensuring that your journey to wellness is a holistic and fulfilling one.

WHY EXERCISING FASTED MAY NOT BE IDEAL FOR WOMEN

Now let us explore why fasted exercise—working out without eating beforehand—can be problematic. While some proponents claim benefits such as increased fat oxidation, the reality is more nuanced, particularly for women. Due to unique hormonal fluctuations, metabolic differences, and energy demands, women may not experience the same benefits from fasted exercise as men. In fact, working out in a fasted state can lead to negative outcomes such as increased stress hormones, reduced performance, and potential long-term metabolic disruptions. This chapter explores why exercising fasted may not be the best choice for women and how to optimize fitness while maintaining energy balance.

The Role of Hormones in Women's Energy Needs

Women's bodies respond differently to fasting and exercise than men's due to the influence of hormones such as estrogen, progesterone, and cortisol. These hormones regulate metabolism, fat storage, and muscle maintenance, making energy balance crucial for optimal performance.

1. **Cortisol and Stress Response**

Fasting and exercise both increase cortisol, the body's primary stress hormone. While some cortisol elevation is normal and even beneficial during exercise, excessive or prolonged spikes can:

- Lead to muscle breakdown instead of muscle growth.
- Increase fat storage, particularly around the midsection.
- Contribute to feelings of fatigue and burnout. For women, fasting before exercise can exacerbate this stress response, making it harder to recover and sustain long-term fitness goals.

2. **Blood Sugar and Energy Levels**

Fasted exercise can lead to low blood sugar levels, causing symptoms such as dizziness, weakness, and brain fog. Women are particularly sensitive to fluctuations in glucose due to differences in insulin response. Inadequate carbohydrate availability before exercise can:

- Decrease endurance and strength.
- Impair cognitive function, affecting focus and motivation.
- Increase cravings later in the day, potentially leading to overeating.

The Impact on Performance and Muscle Growth

Women who exercise fasted may experience a decline in overall workout quality and muscle retention. Key factors to consider include:

1. **Reduced Strength and Endurance**

Studies suggest that consuming a balanced meal or snack before a workout improves strength, endurance, and workout intensity. Fasted exercise, on the other hand, may lead to:

- Decreased power output.
- Increased perception of fatigue.
- Poor recovery post-workout.

2. **Muscle Loss vs. Fat Loss**

While some people believe fasted exercise enhances fat burning, the reality is more complex. Without adequate fuel, the body may break down muscle tissue for energy instead of burning fat. This is particularly concerning for women who already face challenges maintaining muscle mass due to lower testosterone levels compared to men.

The Connection Between Fasted Exercise and Menstrual Health

Fasting and fasted exercise can disrupt hormonal balance, leading to issues such as:

- **Irregular or missing periods (amenorrhea):** Chronic under-fueling signals the body to conserve energy, potentially suppressing reproductive hormones.
- **Thyroid dysregulation:** Insufficient energy intake can slow metabolism and contribute to symptoms such as fatigue and weight gain.
- **Impaired bone health:** Women are already at a higher risk for osteoporosis, and fasted exercise may exacerbate calcium depletion and bone loss.

When Fasted Exercise Might Be Acceptable

While exercising fasted may not be ideal for most women, some may tolerate it under specific conditions:

- **Short, low-intensity sessions:** Walking or gentle yoga may not require pre-workout fueling.
- **Women who feel energized fasting:** Some individuals adapt better than others.
- **Listening to the body:** If energy drops or workouts suffer, eating before exercise is the better choice.

BEST PRACTICES FOR PRE-WORKOUT NUTRITION

To optimize performance and well-being, consider the following pre-exercise nutrition strategies:

1. **Consume a Balanced Pre-Workout Meal or Snack**
    - A mix of protein and carbohydrates, such as Greek yogurt with fruit or a banana with almond butter.
2. **Hydrate Properly**
    - Dehydration exacerbates fatigue and muscle cramps. Drink water before and during workouts.
3. **Experiment with Timing**
    - If a full meal isn't possible, a small snack 30-60 minutes before exercise can still provide benefits.
4. **Prioritize Recovery Nutrition**
    - After exercise, consume a protein-rich meal to aid muscle repair and replenish glycogen stores.

For women, fasted exercise may do more harm than good, leading to increased stress, hormonal imbalances, decreased performance, and potential muscle loss. Instead of prioritizing fasted workouts, focus on nourishing the body with balanced nutrition to enhance strength, endurance, and overall well-being. By fueling workouts properly, women can achieve their fitness goals while maintaining long-term health and energy levels.

SOCIAL AND LIFESTYLE CONSIDERATIONS

Navigating social events while sticking to a fasting schedule can feel like walking a tightrope. There's the allure of good company, the clinking of glasses, and the spread of tempting dishes. Yet, if you're committed to intermittent fasting, these gatherings can become a source of stress. The good news is that with a little planning and a positive mindset, you can enjoy these occasions without derailing your fasting goals. Let's explore how you can maintain your fasting regimen while savoring the joyful moments that social events offer.

MANAGING SOCIAL EVENTS AND DINING OUT WHILE FASTING

A key strategy for managing social events is to align them with your eating windows. When you're in control of the schedule, try to choose events that naturally coincide with the times you're already planning to eat. This makes it easier to participate fully without feeling deprived. For those occasions when you don't have control over timing, consider adjusting your fasting window for the day. Flexibility is your ally here, allowing you to enjoy the event while still maintaining your fasting practice. It's about finding a balance that lets you stay on track with your health goals while also enjoying the company of friends and family.

Communication is another powerful tool. Informing your hosts of your dietary preferences ahead of time can alleviate potential awkwardness. A simple heads-up about your fasting schedule can prompt understanding and support from your hosts. Most people are more than willing to accommodate your needs or at least offer options that fit your dietary approach. Whether it's a request to serve dinner a bit earlier or providing a fasting-friendly snack, open communication can make a significant difference.

When dining out, navigating restaurant menus requires a bit of thought. Focus on selecting menu items that are nutrient-dense and satisfying. Lean proteins, colorful vegetables, and healthy fats are your best friends. Don't hesitate to request modifications to meals, whether it's asking for dressing on the side or substituting a starchy side for a salad. Restaurants are often willing to adapt dishes to meet customer needs, so don't be shy about asking. This ensures you enjoy your meal without compromising your fasting efforts or your enjoyment.

Planning ahead can also be a game-changer. Before heading out, consider eating a small meal if it's close to your fasting window. This can prevent the temptation to overindulge and help you make more mindful choices. Bringing fasting-friendly snacks, like nuts or a piece of fruit, can provide a safety net if you're unsure about the food options available. These snacks can tide you over until you return home, allowing you to stick to your fasting plan without feeling hungry or deprived.

While it's important to maintain your fasting schedule, remember to allow yourself some flexibility. Social interactions are about more than just food. Practicing moderation rather than strict restriction is key. If you decide to indulge a bit more during a special occasion, that's okay. Fasting is a long-term lifestyle choice, not a short-term diet. It's about cultivating habits that fit seamlessly into your life, allowing for the ebb and flow of social events and celebrations.

Focusing on the social experience rather than solely on food can transform your perspective. Engage in conversations, participate in activities, and soak up the atmosphere. These moments are precious and can be enjoyed without the overshadowing concern of breaking your fasting schedule. By shifting the focus from food to connection, you create a more fulfilling experience that aligns with both your social and health goals.

Social Event Planner

Before your next social event, try planning out your approach. List the event details, your fasting window, and any potential challenges. Consider possible menu items and modifications, and note down any snacks you might bring. Reflect on your goals for the event—are you looking to connect with friends, try new foods, or simply enjoy a night out? Use this planner to visualize how you'll incorporate fasting into the event seamlessly, ensuring you can enjoy both your social life and your health journey.

TIME MANAGEMENT TIPS FOR BUSY WOMEN

In the whirlwind of daily life, finding time for fasting-friendly meal preparation can feel like a juggling act. Between work, family, and personal commitments, it's easy to let meal planning slide down the priority list. But with a few strategic tweaks, you can streamline your meal prep, making fasting not just easier but more enjoyable. Batch cooking on weekends is a lifesaver. Spend a few hours preparing large quantities of staples like grains, roasted veggies, or proteins, and store them in the fridge or freezer. When the week gets hectic, you'll have the building blocks for quick, healthy meals ready to go. This method not only saves time but also reduces stress when hunger strikes.

Kitchen gadgets can be your best allies in this endeavor. A slow cooker is especially handy, allowing you to prepare meals with minimal effort. Imagine coming home to the comforting aroma of a hearty stew that's been simmering all day. It's a comforting thought, knowing dinner is ready with just the flick of a switch. Similarly, an instant pot can cut down cooking time significantly, providing you with delicious, nutrient-packed meals without the hassle. These tools can make the process of sticking to your fasting schedule feel less like a chore and more like a well-oiled routine.

Prioritization is key to maintaining balance in your life. Allocating specific times for meal prep and exercise can help create a structure that supports your fasting goals. Consider setting aside a dedicated slot in your calendar for these activities, just as you would for a meeting or appointment. This approach not only ensures that these tasks get done but also helps you approach them with intention rather than as an afterthought. When it comes to fasting, scheduling your windows around work and family commitments can create a rhythm that feels natural and sustainable. If mornings are hectic, consider starting your fasting window later in the day. Find what works for you and adjust as needed, ensuring your fasting routine enhances rather than hinders your lifestyle.

Technology offers a host of tools to enhance time management and make fasting more manageable. Calendar reminders for meal and fasting times can keep you on track, gently nudging you when it's time to switch gears. Meal planning apps like Paprika or

Mealime can eliminate the guesswork, offering recipe ideas and creating shopping lists tailored to your preferences. These apps streamline the process, allowing you to focus on what matters most—nourishing your body and mind. Leveraging these resources can make the logistics of fasting feel less daunting and more like a part of your everyday routine.

Amid the hustle and bustle, self-care often takes a backseat. Yet, it's an integral part of supporting fasting success. Setting aside time for relaxation and hobbies can recharge your spirit and provide a much-needed break from daily demands. Whether it's reading a good book, gardening, or crafting, engaging in activities that bring joy can have a profound impact on your well-being. Mindful breaks during busy days offer moments of calm and reflection, allowing you to reset and refocus. Even a short walk or a few minutes of deep breathing can make a difference. These practices not only support your mental health but also contribute to a more balanced approach to fasting, ensuring you feel nourished in body and soul.

FASTING AND FAMILY: CREATING SUPPORTIVE ENVIRONMENTS

Fasting can sometimes feel like a solitary endeavor, but it doesn't have to be. Involving your family in your fasting routine can be a game changer, turning your personal health goals into a shared experience. Family support is more than just encouragement; it's about creating an environment where your goals are understood and respected. Start by sharing your fasting objectives with your family. Explain what you're trying to achieve, whether it's weight loss, improved energy, or simply better health. Be open about the challenges you might face, such as managing hunger or adjusting meal times. This transparency invites understanding and allows your family to offer the support you need. Encouraging open communication about your needs and challenges can strengthen these relationships, making fasting a collective journey rather than an individual struggle.

Incorporating family preferences into meal planning can make fasting more harmonious. Consider cooking meals that satisfy everyone while still aligning with your fasting goals. This might mean preparing a base meal that's versatile enough for everyone to enjoy, with optional additions for those not fasting. For instance, a hearty vegetable stir-fry can be easily adapted—add a protein source for those who aren't fasting, or serve it over rice for a more filling option. By involving family members in the meal preparation process, you foster a sense of inclusivity. Encourage them to help with meal planning or cooking. Not only does this lighten your load, but it also educates them about your dietary choices and why they're important to you. This shared activity can turn mealtime into a bonding experience where everyone contributes to the table.

Family activities that promote health can further bolster your fasting success. Encourage activities that get everyone moving, like family walks or bike rides. These outings not only promote physical activity but also offer a chance to connect and enjoy each other's company. They're a wonderful way to make exercise feel less like a chore and more like a fun family event. Consider group participation in cooking or nutrition workshops. These can be a great way to learn new recipes and techniques that support your fasting goals. Plus, they provide an opportunity for everyone to learn about health and nutrition in an engaging setting. By turning health into a family affair, you create a supportive environment that benefits everyone involved.

Navigating family gatherings and traditions can be tricky when fasting, but it's entirely possible with a few adjustments.

Modifying traditional recipes to be more fasting-friendly ensures you don't feel left out during family meals. For example, if your family loves a particular pasta dish, consider making a version with zucchini noodles or adding more vegetables to the sauce. This allows you to enjoy the flavors of tradition while staying true to your health goals. Communicating your fasting needs with extended family is important. Let them know about your eating schedule so they can accommodate you where possible. This might mean scheduling meal times a bit earlier or later or ensuring there are options available that fit within your dietary restrictions. Most families are more than happy to support your efforts when they understand your reasoning.

Creating a supportive family environment for fasting is about more than just the food on your plate. It's about cultivating an atmosphere of understanding and collaboration, where your health goals are a priority for everyone. By involving your family in your fasting journey, you build a network of support that encourages success and makes the process more enjoyable. It's a reminder that fasting doesn't have to be a solitary endeavor; it can be a shared experience that brings your family closer together, fostering a collective commitment to health and well-being.

ADAPTING FASTING DURING TRAVEL AND HOLIDAYS

Traveling can throw a wrench into even the most well-oiled fasting routines. You're out of your element, surrounded by new foods and schedules, and that can make sticking to your plan feel like an uphill battle. But with a little foresight, you can keep your fasting regimen on track while still enjoying your adventures. Start by researching meal options and fasting-friendly restaurants before you pack your bags. Many places offer menus that cater to various dietary needs, and a little planning can help you find spots that align with your goals. Look for locations that highlight nutrient-dense dishes, or consider trying cuisines that naturally lend themselves to fasting, such as Mediterranean or Japanese. Knowing where you can find suitable meals in advance saves time and reduces anxiety about where your next meal will come from.

Packing travel-friendly snacks can be a lifesaver. Think of items that are easy to carry and don't require refrigeration, like nuts, seeds, or even dried fruit. These snacks can tide you over during long flights or unexpected delays, ensuring you don't have to compromise on your fasting schedule. They not only stave off hunger but also offer a healthy alternative to the often less-than-ideal options available in airports or on the road. Keeping a few snacks in your bag can provide peace of mind and help you maintain your fasting goals without feeling deprived.

Holidays are another challenge, filled with traditions and meals that don't always align with fasting windows. Flexibility is your ally here. Adjusting your fasting windows to accommodate holiday meals can help you enjoy festive gatherings without guilt. If a big holiday dinner is planned, consider shifting your eating window earlier or later to fit the event. It's about adapting your schedule to fit the occasion, not the other way around. Allowing for special exceptions during holidays is perfectly fine. Remember, fasting is a long-term commitment, and an occasional deviation won't undo your progress. It's about making choices that respect both your health goals and the joy of celebrating with loved ones.

Technology is a powerful tool for maintaining your fasting routine while away from home. Fasting apps can track your eating windows and progress, offering reminders and insights into your habits. This can be particularly helpful when your usual schedule is disrupted. Apps like Zero or FastHabit provide easy-to-use interfaces for tracking fasting periods, helping you stay accountable even when traveling. Fitness trackers can also play a role in maintaining activity levels, offering gentle nudges to keep moving, whether you're sightseeing or lounging by the pool. These tools make it easier to stay on course, providing structure and support when your environment is anything but routine.

Maintaining a positive mindset during travel and holidays is just as important. Embrace flexibility and self-compassion, focusing on the overall picture rather than individual days. It's easy to get caught up in the details, but remembering your broader goals can help keep things in perspective. Practicing gratitude for the experiences and connections you make can shift your focus from what you're missing to what you're gaining. Each meal and moment is part of a larger tapestry, contributing to your ongoing health and happiness.

In the end, fasting is about balance. It's about finding what works for you, even when life throws a curveball. The strategies we've explored—planning meals, packing snacks, using technology, and maintaining a positive mindset—offer a framework for integrating fasting into travel and holidays. These occasions don't have to derail your progress; instead, they can enrich your experience, adding new dimensions to your fasting journey. As we transition from these lifestyle considerations, our next step is to address common concerns and misconceptions, ensuring you're equipped with the knowledge and confidence to navigate fasting with ease.

CASE STUDIES AND SUCCESS STORIES & SOME NOT SO SUCCESSFUL

Have you ever wondered if someone else out there shares your struggle with weight and hormonal balance during menopause? Imagine Sarah, a woman who, much like you, found herself grappling with these exact challenges. Her story is one of transformation and resilience, highlighting the power of listening to your body and embracing change.

CASE STUDY 1: SUCCESS STORY: BALANCING HORMONES AND WEIGHT LOSS

Sarah's journey began with the all-too-familiar trials of menopause. Hot flashes seemed to arrive at the most inconvenient times, leaving her flustered and uncomfortable. Her mood swings felt like a tempest, turning even the simplest interactions into emotional puzzles. Weight gain clung to her midsection despite her sincere efforts with various diets. She felt as though her body had become a stranger, rebelling against her every attempt to regain control. Exercise routines that once left her energized now seemed to drain her, amplifying her frustration. It was as if menopause had thrown a wrench into her body's once well-oiled machine, leaving her feeling powerless and exhausted.

Desperate for a change, Sarah stumbled upon intermittent fasting. Intrigued by the prospect of a structured eating pattern, she decided to give the 16/8 method a try. This meant she would eat within an eight-hour window, from noon to 8 p.m., and fast for the remaining 16 hours. At first, it felt daunting, the idea of skipping breakfast seemed counterintuitive to her previous habits. However, she decided to trust the process, hoping it might offer relief from her menopausal woes. Sarah began incorporating nutrient-dense meals into her eating window, focusing on whole grains, lean proteins, and plenty of vegetables. She found that these foods not only satisfied her hunger but also provided the energy she needed to get through her day.

As the weeks went by, Sarah started to notice subtle changes. The hot flashes that once dictated her day began to wane, becoming less frequent and intense. Her mood swings, too, started to stabilize, allowing her to engage more fully with her family and friends. The weight that seemed immovable gradually began to shift. It wasn't an overnight miracle, but a steady, encouraging decline that boosted her spirits and motivated her to continue. Her energy levels improved as well, making her morning walks something she looked forward to rather than dreaded. Each step felt lighter, not just physically but mentally, as if shedding pounds of worry along with the weight.

Sarah's experience taught her valuable lessons that she's eager to share with you. Patience and consistency became her mantras. She realized that change doesn't happen overnight, and that's okay. By sticking with her fasting schedule and listening to her body's cues, she could adjust her approach as needed. There were days when she felt hungrier than usual, and on those days, she allowed herself to eat a little more, ensuring her meals were still nourishing and balanced. She learned to be gentle with herself, honoring her body's signals rather than fighting against them. This flexibility made all the difference in sustaining her new lifestyle.

Your Personal Fasting Journey

Consider how Sarah's story resonates with your own experiences. Are there aspects of her approach that could inspire changes in your routine? Take a moment to jot down any thoughts or insights you have. This reflection can serve as a roadmap as you explore what works best for your body and lifestyle.

Remember, Sarah's story is just one example of how intermittent fasting can impact life after 50. Every woman's experience is unique, and what worked for her might not be the perfect fit for you. The key is to remain open, curious, and patient with yourself as you embark on your own path to health and vitality.

CASE STUDY 2: OVERCOMING PLATEAUS: HOW ONE WOMAN BROKE THROUGH

You've been on a roll, losing weight steadily and feeling great. But then, out of nowhere, the scale refuses to budge. This is the dreaded weight loss plateau, a familiar roadblock for many on their health journey. At first, everything seems to be going as planned. Pounds drop, your clothes fit better, and you start feeling more energized. But then, seemingly overnight, progress stalls. It's frustrating, demotivating even. The emotional weight of not seeing progress can often feel heavier than the physical weight itself. Our protagonist, Linda, faced this exact challenge.

Linda's initial success with intermittent fasting was like a breath of fresh air. She had lost weight quickly and felt more vibrant than she had in years. But then, the plateau hit. For weeks, despite her best efforts, her weight stayed the same. Linda felt stuck, battling thoughts of doubt and frustration. She knew she needed a change and began exploring new strategies to reignite her progress. One of her first changes was switching from a 16/8 fasting schedule to alternate-day fasting. This method involved fasting every other day, which introduced a new rhythm to her routine and helped shake her body out of its complacency. It wasn't easy at first, but she persisted, hoping this variation would help her break through the stagnation.

In addition to altering her fasting approach, Linda also revamped her exercise routine. She realized that her body had adapted to her usual workouts, so she decided to introduce new forms of exercise. Linda began incorporating strength training and high-intensity interval training (HIIT) into her regimen. These new activities challenged her body in different ways, building muscle and boosting her metabolism. The change was invigorating, providing her with a renewed sense of purpose and motivation. Each session left her feeling stronger and more empowered, adding a positive boost to her mood and mindset.

The most crucial part of Linda's success was her ability to adapt and persevere. She understood that flexibility was key to overcoming her plateau. Experimenting with meal timing and content allowed her to discover what worked best for her body. She played around with different foods, incorporating more protein and fiber to keep her full and energized. Seeking professional guidance from a nutritionist helped refine her approach, offering insights she hadn't considered on her own. This collaboration allowed her to tailor her plan more closely to her needs, ensuring that her efforts were efficient and effective.

Reflecting on her plateau experience, Linda realized how much it taught her about resilience and determination. She came to see the plateau not as a failure but as a natural part of the weight loss process. It was a reminder that bodies adapt and sometimes need a little nudge to continue progressing. Overcoming this challenge gave her newfound confidence, proving that she could tackle obstacles with patience and creativity. Linda's journey through the plateau was transformative, strengthening her resolve and reinforcing her belief in her ability to succeed. Her story is a testament to the power of persistence and the importance of listening to your body and adapting as needed to reach your goals.

CASE STUDY 3: EMBRACING FLEXIBILITY: A JOURNEY TO SUSTAINABLE HEALTH

Meet Margaret, a woman whose life was a whirlwind of commitments. Between her demanding job, family responsibilities, and social engagements, sticking to a rigid fasting schedule felt nearly impossible. She initially tried the 16/8 method, hoping its structure would provide clarity and control. However, it soon became clear that her lifestyle demanded more flexibility. Margaret realized that every day was different—sometimes, she needed to start her day earlier, and other times, family dinners stretched well into the evening. Rather than abandoning fasting altogether, she decided to adapt. She shifted to a more flexible routine, allowing her fasting windows to change based on her daily needs. This adaptability was liberating, transforming fasting from a strict rule into a supportive practice that fit seamlessly into her life.

This newfound flexibility brought unexpected benefits. With less stress around maintaining a rigid schedule, Margaret found her mental well-being improved. She no longer felt guilty for adjusting her fasting window, which reduced the anxiety she associated with eating. This change in mindset made a significant difference, allowing her to enjoy meals with her family without feeling like she was compromising her health goals. Over time, Margaret noticed her adherence to fasting improved. By listening to her body and making adjustments when necessary, she found a rhythm that worked for her, making fasting a sustainable part of her life rather than a fleeting experiment. Her approach became more intuitive, focusing on how she felt each day instead of sticking to a preset schedule.

Margaret's creative solutions to fasting challenges were both practical and inventive. She embraced mindfulness, tuning into her body's signals to determine when she was genuinely hungry. This practice of intuitive eating helped her make more informed choices, guiding her to eat when she needed nourishment and to pause when she was full. During social events, Margaret employed fasting-friendly strategies to stay on track. She would eat a light snack before attending gatherings, ensuring she wasn't ravenous upon arrival. This allowed her to participate in the social aspects of the event without feeling pressured to eat out of hunger. She also discovered that many restaurants offered healthy options, so she didn't feel restricted when dining out. This flexibility became a cornerstone of her success, allowing her to maintain her fasting goals without feeling deprived or isolated.

Reflecting on her journey, Margaret realized that sustainability in fasting and health is rooted in balance and moderation. She learned to prioritize long-term health over short-term results, understanding that quick fixes were often unsustainable. Her focus shifted from immediate weight loss to overall well-being, valuing the small, consistent changes that contributed to her health over time. Embracing this mindset helped her cultivate a positive relationship with food and her body. By letting go of perfectionism, she found peace in knowing that it was okay to have days that didn't go as planned. Balance became her guiding principle, allowing her to enjoy life while still honoring her health goals.

Margaret's story is a testament to the power of flexibility and adaptation in achieving sustainable health. Her journey reminds us that fasting doesn't have to be an all-or-nothing endeavor. It's about finding what works for you, making adjustments along the way, and being kind to yourself in the process. Her experience shows that with patience and creativity, fasting can be a nourishing, enriching part of your life, supporting your health without adding stress or pressure.

CASE STUDY 4: SUSAN'S BATTLE WITH HORMONAL IMBALANCE

At 54, Susan was struggling with weight gain, brain fog, and fatigue. She had recently entered menopause and noticed that no matter how clean she ate or how much she exercised, the scale wouldn't budge. After hearing about the benefits of intermittent fasting, she decided to try the 16:8 method, fasting for 16 hours and eating in an 8-hour window. In the first few weeks, she lost a few pounds and felt lighter, but soon after, she started experiencing increased fatigue, mood swings, and disrupted sleep. A visit to her doctor revealed worsening hormonal imbalances, particularly declining estrogen and elevated cortisol, a stress hormone that can contribute to weight retention and anxiety. Her nutritionist recommended that she transition to a more balanced eating plan with frequent protein-rich meals to support her metabolism and hormonal health. Within a few weeks of implementing these changes, Susan felt more energized, her brain fog improved, and she no longer struggled with erratic mood swings. This experience taught her that fasting-induced stress can negatively impact hormonal balance, making weight management even more challenging for women over 50.

CASE STUDY 5: DIANNE'S STRUGGLE WITH MUSCLE LOSS AND METABOLISM SLOWDOWN

At 63, Dianne wanted to lose 20 pounds to improve her mobility and overall health. She had heard that fasting could help accelerate fat loss, so she decided to adopt an 18:6 fasting schedule while exercising in a fasted state. In the beginning, she noticed the weight coming off quickly, which excited her. However, after two months, she began to feel weaker, experienced frequent muscle cramps, and struggled with joint pain. A DEXA scan revealed that most of her weight loss came from muscle rather than fat. Her body was breaking down muscle tissue for energy because she wasn't consuming enough protein or nutrients to sustain her activity level. As a result, her metabolism slowed, making it even harder to maintain her weight loss. Her trainer recommended she switch to a more frequent eating pattern with adequate protein intake and strength training to rebuild muscle. Within a few months, Dianne regained her strength, felt more energetic, and noticed an improvement in her overall body composition. Her experience showed her that fasting can contribute to muscle loss, making long-term weight management more difficult for aging women.

CASE STUDY 6: MARIA'S BLOOD SUGAR ROLLERCOASTER

Maria, 57, was diagnosed with prediabetes and wanted to manage her blood sugar naturally. She decided to try alternate-day fasting, believing it would improve her insulin sensitivity. On fasting days, she ate very little, and when she did eat, she often consumed carbohydrate-heavy meals, thinking she needed quick energy. However, instead of stabilizing her blood sugar, she started experiencing extreme highs and lows, leading to dizziness, irritability, and constant sugar cravings. Her glucose monitor showed erratic blood sugar spikes, and she often felt fatigued throughout the day.

Concerned about these fluctuations, she consulted a dietitian who advised her to switch to a balanced diet with meals every 4-5 hours, incorporating protein, fiber, and healthy fats to maintain steady blood sugar levels. After making these adjustments, Maria's blood sugar readings stabilized, her energy levels improved, and she no longer felt the intense hunger and cravings that fasting had triggered. This experience highlighted the potential risks of fasting for women with blood sugar issues and reinforced the importance of a steady, well-balanced diet over extreme dietary restrictions.

COMMUNITY SUPPORT: FINDING MOTIVATION IN OTHERS

Have you ever noticed how a shared laugh or a nod of understanding can make a world of difference? For many women, the journey through menopause and weight management can feel like a solitary battle. But what if it didn't have to be that way? Many have found solace and strength in the arms of a community. Take for instance, the story of Janet, who felt overwhelmed by the changes her body was enduring. She stumbled upon an online fasting group and decided to join, hoping to find some guidance and support. What she found was so much more—a sisterhood of understanding women who were walking the same path.

In these groups, Janet found a haven of shared experiences. There were daily check-ins where members would share their victories and struggles, creating a space where accountability thrived. The encouragement she received from other women was uplifting. It wasn't just about sharing numbers on a scale; it was about celebrating small victories, like resisting that late-night snack or completing a fast without feeling fatigued. These interactions gave Janet the motivation to keep going, knowing she wasn't alone. It was in this supportive bubble that she truly began to flourish, finding new ways to challenge herself and grow.

Janet also attended local wellness workshops and seminars. These gatherings allowed her to meet like-minded individuals face-to-face, strengthening her resolve. The workshops were more than just informative sessions; they were opportunities to forge real connections. Surrounded by women who understood her journey, Janet felt a renewed sense of purpose. The advice and tips shared by others enriched her own experience, offering fresh perspectives and solutions she hadn't considered before. Attending these events became a cornerstone of her routine, giving her the tools she needed to continue her fasting journey with confidence.

The mentorship she received within these communities was invaluable. Experienced fasters were more than willing to share their wisdom, offering guidance on everything from meal planning to overcoming cravings. Janet learned from their success stories, discovering new fasting techniques and adjustments that could better fit her lifestyle. The peer learning aspect of the community was a treasure trove of information, allowing her to tailor her approach and avoid common pitfalls. This collective knowledge empowered her to make informed decisions, injecting her fasting routine with the vigor it needed to be sustainable.

The empowerment Janet felt from being part of a community was profound. It wasn't just about the weight loss or the health benefits—though those were significant. It was about the confidence she gained from participating in a collective journey. Building friendships and support networks gave her a sense of belonging that transcended the physical changes she was experiencing. These relationships became a source of strength, encouraging her to push through challenging times and celebrate her achievements, no matter how small.

In this chapter, we've explored how community can transform your fasting experience, providing the support and encouragement needed to persevere. As you consider your own journey, remember that you don't have to go it alone. There's a world of support out there waiting to guide you, inspire you, and celebrate with you. In the next chapter, we will explore the holistic approach to health, looking at how you can integrate fasting with other lifestyle changes to enhance your overall well-being.

EMBRACING A HOLISTIC APPROACH TO HEALTH

Have you ever felt like life is pulling you in a thousand different directions, leaving you little time to focus on yourself? Taking care of our health often feels like another task on the to-do list, yet it doesn't have to be that way. What if embracing a holistic approach to health could transform not just your body but your mind and spirit, too? This chapter focuses on the holistic wellness that lies at the heart of long-term health for women over 50. Let's explore how practices like mindfulness and meditation can become invaluable tools in this journey, helping you find peace amidst the chaos, soothe anxiety, and enhance your overall well-being.

THE POWER OF MINDFULNESS AND MEDITATION

Mindfulness and meditation have become buzzwords in the wellness world, but their benefits go far beyond the trend. These practices invite you to slow down and truly be present, offering a refuge from the fast-paced demands of daily life. Mindfulness involves focusing your attention on the present moment and observing your thoughts and sensations without judgment. Scientific studies, like those conducted by the Mayo Clinic, suggest that mindfulness can ease menopausal symptoms, reducing irritability, anxiety, and depression (SOURCE 1). This calming effect is crucial for managing the stress and anxiety that often accompany this phase of life. Mindfulness and meditation can enhance focus and cognitive function, sharpening your mental clarity and improving your ability to handle life's challenges with grace and composure. Imagine navigating your day with greater ease, free from the mental clutter that often weighs you down.

Incorporating mindfulness into daily life doesn't have to be daunting. It can be as simple as taking a few moments each day for mindful breathing exercises. Find a quiet spot, close your eyes, and take a deep breath in through your nose, letting your belly expand. Hold for a moment, then exhale slowly through your mouth. This simple act of focusing on your breath can help you relax and center yourself, even during the busiest of days. Another effective technique is the body scan meditation, where you mentally "scan" your body from head to toe, noticing any tension or discomfort. This practice increases awareness of your physical state, encouraging you to release tension and foster a sense of calm and relaxation.

Mindfulness can significantly enhance your fasting experiences, making them more fulfilling and less challenging. By cultivating patience and presence during fasting, you learn to listen to your body's needs and respond with kindness. Meditation can help manage cravings and hunger, shifting your focus from the discomfort of an empty stomach to the richness of the present moment. When hunger strikes, try a brief meditation session to redirect your thoughts and reinforce your commitment to your health goals. This shift in perspective can transform fasting from a test of willpower into an opportunity for self-discovery and growth.

Developing a personal meditation practice tailored to your needs can be an enriching endeavor. Begin by setting aside a specific time each day for meditation, allowing it to become a cherished part of your routine. Whether it's first thing in the morning to set a positive tone for the day or in the evening to unwind, consistency is key. Explore different meditation styles to find what resonates with you, whether it's guided meditation with a soothing voice leading the way or silent meditation where you immerse yourself in the tranquility of stillness. The beauty of meditation is that there's no one right way to do it—it's about finding what feels right for you.

Creating Your Meditation Space

Let's create a personal sanctuary for your meditation practice. Choose a quiet spot in your home where you feel comfortable and at ease. Add elements that inspire serenity, like a soft cushion, a cozy blanket, or a few scented candles. Consider playing gentle music or nature sounds to enhance the atmosphere. This space will serve as your retreat—a place where you can retreat to daily, even if only for a few moments, to nurture your mind and spirit.

STRESS MANAGEMENT TECHNIQUES FOR BETTER HEALTH

Stress is that unwelcome guest who arrives uninvited and overstays its welcome. It affects every part of your life, including your health and fasting goals. When you're stressed, your body releases cortisol, the stress hormone, which can wreak havoc on your metabolism and lead to weight gain, especially around your midsection. Ever notice how, during stressful times, reaching for comfort foods seems almost automatic? That's because emotional eating is a common response to stress. It's a coping mechanism that provides temporary relief but can undermine your fasting efforts and overall well-being. Recognizing the impact of stress on your health is the first step toward regaining control.

To effectively manage stress and its impact on your life, explore a variety of stress management techniques that promote relaxation. Progressive muscle relaxation is a wonderful tool that can help release physical tension. It involves tensing and then relaxing each muscle group in your body, starting from your toes and working your way up to your head. This practice not only eases physical tension but also calms the mind. Another helpful technique is journaling, which allows you to process your emotions by putting them on paper. It's like having a heart-to-heart with yourself, helping you understand and work through your feelings. Writing down your thoughts and worries can provide clarity and relief, making it easier to let go of stressors.

Consistency is key when it comes to stress management. Creating a daily stress relief routine helps integrate these practices into your life, making them as natural as brushing your teeth. Whether it's dedicating ten minutes in the morning to stretching or ending your day with a few pages in your journal, regular practice builds resilience against stress. Incorporating stress management into your everyday activities can be as simple as taking a few deep breaths while waiting at a red light or enjoying a quiet cup of tea without distractions. These small moments of calm can accumulate, gradually reducing your overall stress levels.

Don't be afraid to explore creative activities that bring you joy and relaxation. Engaging in artistic pursuits like painting or crafting can be incredibly therapeutic, offering a way to express yourself and unwind. Even if you're not the next Picasso, the act of creating something with your hands can be deeply satisfying. Spending time in nature is another powerful stress reliever. Whether it's a leisurely walk in the park, gardening, or simply sitting outside and listening to the birds, nature has a unique way of rejuvenating the spirit. It provides a peaceful backdrop that encourages you to slow down and breathe.

Stress Management Checklist

Consider creating a checklist of stress management activities that resonate with you. Keep it somewhere visible, like on your fridge or desk, as a reminder to incorporate these practices into your life. Include both quick fixes and longer activities, ensuring you have a variety of tools at your disposal for different situations. This checklist serves as a handy guide, helping you stay committed to your stress management routine and supporting your health and fasting goals.

SLEEP OPTIMIZATION: ENHANCING REST AND RECOVERY

Have you ever tossed and turned, wondering why sleep seems so elusive just when you need it most? You're not alone. Sleep plays a critical role in every aspect of our health, and for women over 50, getting quality rest is crucial not just for feeling refreshed but for maintaining hormonal balance and supporting fasting efforts. Sleep impacts hormone regulation profoundly. It's during those deep, rejuvenating slumbers that your body releases growth hormones and regulates cortisol, the stress hormone. This intricate dance affects your metabolism, influencing how energy is stored and used. Lack of sleep can throw this balance off, leading to weight gain and increased cravings, both of which can derail your fasting goals. Your brain also needs sleep to function at its best. Good sleep enhances cognitive abilities, sharpens focus, and improves memory. Think of it as hitting the reset button for your mind, clearing away the fog, and helping you tackle each day with clarity and vigor.

Improving sleep quality is a goal worth pursuing, and small adjustments can yield big results. Establishing a consistent sleep schedule is one of the most effective ways to ensure a good night's rest. Going to bed and waking up at the same time each day, even on weekends, helps regulate your body's internal clock. Over time, this consistency cues your body to feel sleepy and wakeful at the right times. Creating a calming bedtime routine can also signal your body that it's time to wind down. This could include activities like reading a book, listening to soothing music, or indulging in a warm bath. Avoiding screens an hour before bed is essential, as the blue light emitted by phones and computers can interfere with the production of melatonin, the sleep hormone.

Many of us face common sleep disturbances that disrupt our rest. Insomnia, characterized by difficulty falling or staying asleep, can be managed with relaxation techniques. Gentle yoga or stretching before bed can relax your muscles and mind, preparing you for sleep. If you're prone to waking up during the night, dietary adjustments might help. Consuming lighter meals in the evening and avoiding caffeine or alcohol close to bedtime can reduce nighttime awakenings. It's also worth experimenting with herbal teas, like chamomile or valerian root, known for their sleep-promoting properties.

Evaluating and optimizing your sleep environment can further enhance your rest. Your bedroom should be a sanctuary of calm and comfort. Start by using blackout curtains to block any unwanted light, creating a dark environment conducive to sleep. Consider investing in a quality mattress and pillows that support your body comfortably. Maintaining a cool room temperature is also key, as a cooler room can promote deeper sleep. Aim for a temperature that feels refreshing rather than chilly. Incorporate soothing elements like an essential oil diffuser or a white noise machine to drown out disruptive sounds. These small tweaks can transform your bedroom into a haven for restful sleep, making it easier for you to drift off and stay asleep.

Sleep isn't just an escape from the day; it's an integral part of your health and well-being. Prioritizing sleep means prioritizing yourself and recognizing that rest is a foundation for all other aspects of health, including successful fasting. By making intentional changes to your sleep habits and environment, you create a nurturing space for your body to recharge, ensuring you're ready to greet each new day with energy and enthusiasm.

BUILDING A HOLISTIC WELLNESS ROUTINE

Picture your wellness routine as a vibrant tapestry woven from threads of physical activity, nutrition, and mindfulness. Each element contributes its own color and texture, creating a balanced and beautiful whole. Physical activity is more than just exercise; it's about movement that feels joyful and sustainable. Whether it's a brisk walk, a dance class, or gentle yoga, find what makes you feel alive and incorporate it regularly. Nutrition is another crucial strand, not just about what you eat but how you nourish your body. Focus on whole foods that fuel your body and support your health goals. And mindfulness, that ever-important practice of being present, ties it all together, helping you stay connected to your body and mind. Together, these components form the foundation of a holistic wellness routine, supporting not just your physical health but your mental and emotional well-being as well.

Creating a personalized wellness plan is about aligning your routine with your individual needs and goals. Start by setting realistic and achievable objectives. Maybe it's increasing your daily steps, trying a new healthy recipe each week, or dedicating time to a hobby that brings you joy. Write these goals down, and remember to track your progress. Keeping a journal or using an app can help you see how far you've come and identify areas where you might need to adjust. It's not about perfection; it's about creating a routine that feels right for you. Be flexible, and don't be afraid to tweak your plan as your needs change. Your wellness routine should evolve with you, adapting to the ebbs and flows of life.

Balance and flexibility are key to maintaining a successful wellness routine. It's important to allow for adaptation in your schedule. Life is unpredictable and sometimes plans change. Maybe you skip a workout one day or indulge in a treat that wasn't on the menu. That's okay. The key is to return to your routine without guilt, recognizing the importance of rest and downtime. Your body and mind need these breaks to recharge and come back stronger. By embracing balance, you give yourself the grace to enjoy life while still prioritizing your health. It's a dance between discipline and freedom, where both can coexist harmoniously.

As you continue on this path, don't forget to celebrate your achievements. Acknowledging your progress is a powerful motivator and can reinforce positive habits. Reflect on your growth and the changes you've made, no matter how small. Maybe you've noticed more energy, better sleep, or a more positive outlook. Whatever it is, take time to appreciate these victories. Engage in self-care activities as rewards for your hard work. Treat yourself to a relaxing bath, a new book, or a leisurely day in nature. These moments of celebration remind you that wellness is not just a destination but a way of life.

In weaving together these elements, you're crafting a wellness routine that's uniquely yours. Each choice you make contributes to a healthier, more balanced life, empowering you to face each day with vitality and purpose. Remember, the journey of wellness is a continuous one, filled with learning and growth. As you embrace this holistic approach, you'll find that the changes you make ripple outwards, enhancing not just your health but your entire life.

SELF-COMPASSION AND BODY POSITIVITY

Have you ever noticed how you speak to yourself when you're having a tough day? If you're like many, that inner voice can be surprisingly harsh, quick to criticize, and slow to forgive. Now, imagine if you could turn that voice into one of your biggest cheerleaders, offering kindness and understanding instead. This is where self-compassion comes in, acting as a powerful tool for mental well-being, especially during the whirlwind of changes that come with aging and menopause. Think of it as a comforting friend who's always there, reminding you that you're doing your best and that it's okay to stumble along the way.

Incorporating self-compassion into your health journey isn't just a feel-good exercise. It plays a crucial role in reducing self-criticism and fostering a kinder internal dialogue. When you practice self-compassion, you allow yourself to make mistakes without the heavy burden of guilt or shame. This shift can enhance emotional resilience, helping you bounce back from setbacks more quickly and with greater ease. Research shows that self-compassion can lead to more positive thoughts and responses to challenges, which can significantly boost your overall well-being (SOURCE 1). By treating yourself with the same kindness you would offer a friend, you create a supportive environment where growth and healing can flourish.

So, how can you start practicing self-compassion daily? One practical approach is to incorporate self-compassionate affirmations or mantras into your routine. These affirmations can be as simple as reminding yourself, "I am enough," or "It's okay to take things one step at a time." By repeating these phrases, you reinforce a positive and nurturing mindset, gradually replacing criticism with understanding. Another powerful tool is journaling. Taking a few minutes each day to reflect on your experiences and emotions can foster self-awareness and acceptance. Write about your challenges, but also celebrate your strengths and achievements. This practice can illuminate patterns and guide you toward a more compassionate view of yourself.

Acceptance plays a vital role in navigating personal challenges. It involves acknowledging and embracing imperfections, understanding that they are a natural part of being human. Instead of battling against difficulties, acceptance allows you to see them as opportunities for growth and learning. This mindset encourages you to approach challenges with curiosity and patience rather than frustration or defeat. By reframing obstacles in this way, you empower yourself to navigate life's ups and downs with grace and resilience.

Cultivating a compassionate mindset requires ongoing effort and intention. It starts with practicing active listening and empathy with yourself. Pay attention to your thoughts and feelings without judgment, recognizing that everyone experiences difficult emotions and moments of self-doubt. By showing empathy to yourself, you create a safe space for healing and transformation. Engaging in mindfulness activities can further support this process. Activities like meditation or yoga promote self-awareness, helping you connect with your body and mind in a nonjudgmental way. These practices encourage you to be present, to feel what you're feeling, and to accept yourself just as you are.

Self-Compassion Journal Prompt

Consider setting aside a few minutes each day to write about a moment when you were hard on yourself. Reflect on how you might respond differently with kindness and understanding. What would you say to a friend in the same situation? Use this exercise to practice self-compassion and transform your inner dialogue into one of support and empathy. By doing so, you'll nurture a more compassionate relationship with yourself, one that celebrates your journey and honors your unique path to wellness.

REDEFINING SUCCESS: BEYOND THE SCALE

Have you ever stepped on the scale only to find that the number staring back at you dictates your mood for the rest of the day? It's time to rethink that narrative. For too long, we've been conditioned to view weight as the ultimate indicator of health. But isn't it time we challenged this outdated notion? Health is so much more than a number—it's about how you feel, your energy levels, and your mental well-being. Consider the concept of non-scale victories, those moments when your clothes fit better, your energy soars, or you simply feel good in your skin. These victories speak to a deeper sense of wellness that transcends the digits on a scale. They remind us that success in health is multifaceted, encompassing various aspects of our lives.

Let's talk about setting goals that reflect this broader understanding of health. Imagine focusing on personal growth, where achievements are measured not just in pounds lost but in strength gained and happiness found. Picture yourself setting goals that celebrate physical strength and endurance—like lifting a heavier weight, running a bit further, or dancing without getting winded. These milestones can bring incredible satisfaction and are often more sustainable than weight loss alone. Then there's the emotional side of things. By setting intentions for emotional balance and stress reduction, you give yourself permission to prioritize mental health as much as physical health. This might mean developing coping strategies for stress or dedicating time to relax and recharge. These goals, though different from traditional measures, play a crucial role in achieving a holistic sense of well-being.

Think about individuals who have redefined what success means on their health journeys. Take Mary, for example, who decided to focus on increased stamina and physical mobility after feeling restricted by her previous goals centered solely on weight. As she began to walk more and gain endurance, she realized the joy and satisfaction that came with moving her body freely. Her newfound energy and agility became her markers of success rather than the numbers on a scale. There's also David, who found happiness in cultivating healthy habits, like preparing nutritious meals and enjoying them with family. His understanding of success evolved to include the pleasure of these shared moments and the nourishment they provided, both physically and emotionally.

Changing how we define success can have a profound impact on motivation and sustainability. By cultivating a growth mindset, we learn to view challenges as opportunities to learn and improve rather than setbacks to be feared. This mindset fosters resilience, allowing us to stay committed to our health pursuits even when progress feels slow. Embracing the process, rather than fixating on outcomes, can transform how we approach our goals. It encourages us to appreciate each step as part of a larger journey full of learning, growth, and self-discovery. This shift in perspective not only enhances our motivation but also makes our path to health more enjoyable and rewarding.

As you begin to redefine success in your own health journey, remember that it's a deeply personal endeavor. What matters most is how you feel in your body and your life. Whether it's the joy of a morning walk, the peace of mind from a good night's sleep, or the strength found in lifting your grandchild, these are the victories that truly count. So, let's celebrate all the ways we can thrive beyond the scale and beyond the numbers.

CELEBRATING SMALL WINS AND PROGRESS

Have you ever noticed how a small pat on the back can make a huge difference? That's the magic of celebrating those little victories along your health journey. Recognizing incremental achievements isn't just about giving yourself a gold star; it's about fueling the fire within you to keep going. When you acknowledge improvements in your fitness levels or dietary habits, you're reinforcing your commitment to a healthier lifestyle. Perhaps you've noticed that climbing stairs no longer leaves you breathless, or your favorite jeans fit just a bit better. These are not minor details —they're milestones on your path to better health. Consistently sticking to a fasting schedule, despite the temptations of social gatherings or the lure of late-night snacks, is another achievement worth applauding. Each day you stay true to your goals is a testament to your resilience and dedication.

So, how can you creatively celebrate these wins? Consider planning a self-care day as a reward for your hard work. Whether it's a long soak in the bath, a spa treatment, or simply a quiet afternoon with a good book, taking time to pamper yourself is a powerful way to acknowledge your progress. Treating yourself to a new hobby-related item or a book you've wanted to read can also serve as a tangible reminder of your accomplishments. These rewards don't have to be extravagant; they just need to be meaningful to you. It's about recognizing your efforts and giving yourself the credit you deserve.

Keeping track of your progress is crucial, and a dedicated journal or diary can be an invaluable tool. Documenting your health milestones allows you to see how far you've come and provides motivation during tougher times. You might choose to jot down weekly reflections, noting any positive changes or challenges you've faced. Visual reminders, such as mood boards or charts, can also help you stay focused on your goals. Seeing your progress laid out visually can be incredibly satisfying and motivating. These tools not only keep you accountable but also serve as a personal record of your journey, one that you can look back on with pride.

Positive reinforcement plays a significant role in sustaining change. Sharing your successes with supportive friends or family can amplify your achievements, providing a sense of community and encouragement. Celebrating together can strengthen bonds and remind you that you're not alone in your pursuits. Engaging in community celebrations or challenges can also be invigorating. Whether it's participating in a local fun run or joining an online group dedicated to a shared health goal, these experiences foster a sense of belonging and collective motivation. They remind you that your efforts are part of a larger tapestry of shared experiences and aspirations.

Recognizing and celebrating these small wins is not about vanity or self-indulgence. It's about building a foundation of positivity and self-worth that supports your ongoing health endeavors. Each step forward, no matter how small, is a step towards a healthier, more fulfilling life. By taking the time to acknowledge and celebrate your progress, you reinforce the healthy behaviors that will carry you forward. It's about creating a cycle of motivation and success, where each victory propels you to strive for the next. So, give yourself a little credit—you've earned it.

DEVELOPING A POSITIVE BODY IMAGE

In a world where media often dictates what beauty should look like, it's easy to feel like you're constantly falling short. Every day, we're bombarded with images of youth and so-called perfection, creating unrealistic standards that can deeply affect how we see ourselves. The media's portrayal of aging as something to be feared rather than celebrated doesn't help either. It's no wonder many of us struggle with body image issues, feeling pressured to fit a mold that was never designed with us in mind. Cultural expectations about body shape and size further complicate this, adding layers of stress and self-doubt. These ideals often ignore the natural changes that come with age, leaving us to question our worth based on appearance alone. But here's the truth: Your worth isn't tied to how closely you resemble a magazine cover. It's about embracing who you are and the story your body tells.

Building a positive body image starts with gratitude. Take a moment to appreciate what your body does for you daily. The simple act of breathing, moving, and experiencing life is nothing short of miraculous. By focusing on your body's abilities rather than its appearance, you shift the narrative from criticism to appreciation. Engaging in activities that foster body appreciation can also be transformative. Yoga, for example, connects you with your body in a gentle, respectful way, encouraging you to listen and respond to its needs. Dance, too, is a celebration of movement and freedom, allowing you to express yourself without judgment. These practices remind you that your body is more than just a shell; it's a vessel for joy, strength, and resilience.

Surrounding yourself with positivity is crucial in nurturing body confidence. Curating your social media feeds to include body-positive content can make a significant difference. Follow accounts that celebrate diversity and inclusivity, showcasing real people with real stories. This shift in what you consume visually can alter your self-perception, helping you see the beauty in variation and authenticity. Building a network of body-positive individuals and communities provides a support system where encouragement and acceptance are the norms. These connections can uplift you, reinforcing the belief that you are valuable just as you are.

Embracing your individuality and self-expression is another powerful way to enhance body image. Exploring fashion and beauty as forms of self-expression allows you to experiment and have fun with your appearance. It's about wearing what makes you feel good, not what society dictates. Perhaps it's a bold lipstick that makes you feel powerful or a cozy sweater that wraps you in comfort. Celebrating diversity in body types and appearances helps you recognize the beauty in uniqueness, fostering an environment where differences are cherished rather than criticized. When you embrace your individuality, you're not just accepting your body; you're celebrating it.

Our bodies are canvases of our experiences, change, and growth. They carry us through life's ups and downs, adapting and evolving as we do. By cultivating gratitude, surrounding ourselves with positivity, and expressing our individuality, we forge a path to a more positive body image. This journey isn't about striving for an ideal but about finding peace and pride in who you are. As we move forward, let's continue to explore how these concepts can influence other areas of our lives, creating a ripple effect of confidence and self-love.

TOOLS AND RESOURCES FOR CONTINUED SUCCESS

TECHNOLOGY AT YOUR SERVICE

Have you ever wished for a personal assistant to guide you through your health journey, especially during the ups and downs of fasting and menopause? Technology, in many ways, can serve that role, offering not just convenience but also a sense of empowerment. In today's digital age, we have access to a plethora of tools that can make managing your health easier and more efficient. From apps that track your fasting windows to gadgets that monitor your physical activity, these technologies serve as allies in your pursuit of a balanced, healthy lifestyle.

Technology can be a game-changer when it comes to fasting, especially for women over 50 navigating the complexities of menopause. Apps designed specifically for fasting provide real-time tracking, helping you manage your eating and fasting periods with greater ease. They offer detailed insights into your dietary habits and nutrient intake, allowing you to make informed decisions about what to eat during your eating windows. With just a few taps on your smartphone, you can view your fasting schedule, monitor your progress, and adjust your plans as needed. This level of convenience and insight can be incredibly motivating, offering a clear picture of your efforts and successes.

Among the popular fasting apps available, Zero and FastHabit stand out for their intuitive tracking features. Zero offers a simple interface that lets you start and stop your fasts with ease while providing insights into your fasting habits and progress over time. FastHabit, on the other hand, allows you to customize fasting goals and reminders, making it easier to stick to your chosen routine. For those looking to track their nutritional intake alongside fasting, MyFitnessPal is an excellent choice. It offers comprehensive nutritional logging, helping you keep tabs on calories, macros, and micronutrients, ensuring you meet your dietary needs even while fasting.

Wearable gadgets have also become essential tools for health monitoring, offering valuable metrics that enhance accountability. Fitness trackers like Fitbit can monitor your physical activity, heart rate, and even sleep patterns, providing a holistic view of your health. These devices help you stay active and encourage you to move more, which is crucial for maintaining muscle mass and overall well-being as you age. Smart scales add another layer of insight, tracking not just weight but also body composition changes, such as fat and muscle percentage. This data can be particularly motivating, as it shows progress beyond what the scale alone can reveal.

Experimenting with different technologies can help you find the best fit for your personal needs and preferences. Testing different app features can reveal which ones align with your user-friendliness requirements, ensuring that the technology enhances rather than complicates your health journey. Exploring gadgets that align with your specific health goals can also be rewarding. Whether you aim to increase physical activity, improve sleep quality, or optimize your nutritional intake, there's likely a tool out there that can support you.

Technology Trial Checklist

Consider creating a checklist to guide you through trying new fasting apps and health gadgets. List features that are important to you, such as ease of use, data tracking, and community support. As you test each tool, note what works and what doesn't. This hands-on approach can help you make informed decisions about which technologies best fit your lifestyle and health goals.

Incorporating technology into your health routine can make fasting and managing menopause not only more manageable but also more enjoyable. These tools provide structure, insight, and motivation, helping you stay on track and achieve your health goals with confidence. By embracing these digital allies, you can navigate the challenges of fasting and menopause with ease and empowerment.

FINDING EXPERT GUIDANCE: COACHES AND HEALTH PROFESSIONALS

When you're navigating the challenges of menopause and trying to adopt a fasting regimen, having a professional by your side can make all the difference. Think of expert guidance as a personalized toolbox filled with tailored advice and encouragement designed just for you. Health professionals can craft nutrition and fitness plans that align with your body's unique needs and goals. They provide insights into how fasting might affect you personally and suggest adaptations that can enhance your results. This kind of customized support not only empowers you but also helps you stay motivated and informed.

Choosing the right coach or health professional is crucial for your success. Start by verifying their credentials and experience in the relevant fields. You want someone who understands both the science and the practicalities of fasting, especially as it relates to women over 50. Look for certifications from reputable organizations, and don't be shy about asking potential coaches about their qualifications. Testimonials or reviews from previous clients can offer valuable insights into their effectiveness and style. Personal recommendations from friends or family who have had positive experiences can also guide you to the right expert.

There's a wide range of professional support available, each with its own strengths. Nutritionists and dietitians are fantastic for dietary advice. They can help you develop meal plans that not only support fasting but also cater to any specific dietary needs or preferences you might have. If exercise is a key focus, fitness trainers are invaluable. They can design personalized exercise programs that work in harmony with your fasting schedule, ensuring you maintain muscle mass and energy levels. Then there are health coaches who take a more holistic approach, offering lifestyle coaching that addresses not just diet and exercise but also stress management and overall well-being.

Once you've chosen a professional, open communication is the cornerstone of effective support. Be clear about your health goals and any concerns you have. Whether it's managing weight, improving energy, or addressing specific menopausal symptoms, sharing these details helps your coach tailor their guidance to your needs. Regular updates on your progress and challenges ensure that the support you receive remains relevant and effective. Don't hesitate to voice any difficulties or adjustments you feel are necessary. This dialogue not only enhances your experience but also fosters a trusting and collaborative relationship.

Working with a professional can feel like having a trusted cheerleader in your corner. They provide not just knowledge but also the motivation to keep pushing forward, even when the going gets tough. Their expertise and encouragement can transform your approach to health, making it more structured and achievable. So, if you're considering enlisting expert help, know that it's more than just a step in the right direction—it's a leap towards a healthier, more empowered you.

CREATING A PERSONALIZED HEALTH JOURNAL

Imagine having a space where you can spill your thoughts, track your progress, and even vent a little on those tougher days. That's what a health journal can become for you—a trusted companion on your health path. Keeping a journal offers more than just a record of your meals or fasting windows; it's a tool for enhancing self-awareness. As you jot down daily experiences and reflections, you gain insights into how different fasting methods affect your mood, energy levels, and even physical changes. This practice can help you connect the dots between what you eat, how you fast, and how you feel. It's like having a conversation with yourself, where you can explore what works and what doesn't, all in one place.

Setting up a health journal can be both fun and personal. Consider structuring it with sections dedicated to meal and fasting logs, where you can note what you ate, how long you fasted, and how you felt afterward. This can help you see patterns over time, such as which foods leave you energized or sluggish. Another section could be for goal setting and achievement tracking. Write down your health goals—whether it's losing weight, maintaining energy, or managing menopause symptoms—and track your progress.

Seeing your achievements, no matter how small, can be incredibly motivating. It's like having a personal cheerleader in your corner, reminding you of how far you've come.

To make journaling more engaging, try incorporating creative techniques. Visual elements like charts and graphs can transform your data into a more digestible and visually appealing format. You might use a graph to track your weight or a chart to monitor your mood fluctuations over time. These visuals not only make the information easier to understand but also offer a quick snapshot of your progress. Prompts can also encourage deeper self-exploration and reflection. Questions like "What am I grateful for today?" or "What challenges did I overcome this week?" can guide you to insights that might not surface in your day-to-day thoughts.

Consistency is key in journaling, much like with any healthy habit. Setting aside a specific time each day to write can help make it a regular part of your routine. Whether it's first thing in the morning with your coffee or at night as you wind down, find a time that feels right for you. This dedicated time allows you to reflect on the day, review your entries, and identify patterns or insights that might otherwise go unnoticed. Over time, you might notice how certain foods affect your energy or how stress impacts your fasting efforts. These observations can be invaluable in making informed decisions about your health.

Sample Journal Layout

A sample journal layout might include a two-page spread with the left page for daily logs and the right page for reflections and goal tracking. On the left, jot down meals, fasting windows, and any symptoms or moods. On the right, reflect on what went well and what could be improved, and set intentions for the next day. This layout can help you organize your thoughts and keep your journal entries structured and purposeful.

The beauty of a health journal is its adaptability. It grows with you, reflecting your evolving needs and goals. It becomes a record not just of your health but of your resilience and growth. By making journaling a regular practice, you create a space where you can explore, reflect, and celebrate.

BUILDING A SUPPORT NETWORK FOR ACCOUNTABILITY

Think about your closest friends - the ones who text you, "How'd that doctor's appointment go?" or notice when you've been drinking more water lately. That's what real support looks like. It's the friend who says, "Hey, want to go for a walk?" on a day when you'd rather stay on the couch or the family member who learns to cook healthier meals alongside you.

Having people in your corner changes everything. Maybe it's the colleague who brings an extra healthy snack to share or your walking buddy who shows up even on rainy days. These connections matter because let's face it - some days you wake up and just don't feel like sticking to your health goals. But knowing your sister is waiting for you at the gym, or your friend is counting on you for that morning run... that gets you moving.

Plus, there's something powerful about swapping stories with others who get it. Maybe they've found a great way to meal prep that you hadn't thought of, or they understand exactly why that 3 PM sugar craving is so tough to beat. When you're feeling frustrated or celebrating a win, these are the people who truly understand because they've been there, too.

Creating or joining a support group can be a game-changer. With the rise of digital communication, online forums, and social media groups have blossomed into vibrant communities where fasting enthusiasts gather to share tips and stories. These platforms offer the convenience of connecting with people worldwide, each bringing unique insights and encouragement. For those who prefer face-to-face interactions, local fitness or wellness meetups provide a personal touch. Meeting in person allows for deeper connections and the opportunity to engage in activities together, whether it's a group walk, a cooking class, or a meditation session. These gatherings foster a sense of belonging and community, which are vital elements in sustaining motivation.

Accountability partners can be particularly effective. These one-on-one relationships offer personalized support and enhance commitment. By setting joint goals and check-in schedules, you and your partner hold each other accountable. This dynamic creates a powerful incentive to stick to your plans. Together, you celebrate successes and navigate setbacks, turning challenges into shared victories. The bond formed through this partnership can be incredibly motivating as you witness each other's progress and growth.

Fostering a positive and supportive environment is essential for these networks to thrive. Surrounding yourself with encouraging and understanding individuals creates a space where you feel safe to share your journey. It's important to share resources and tips within the network, as this collective knowledge can be invaluable. Whether it's a new recipe, a motivational podcast, or a book that inspired you, sharing these resources enriches the group and fosters a culture of generosity and support. Creating a safe space for open discussions allows everyone to express their thoughts and feelings without fear of judgment, enhancing trust and camaraderie.

The beauty of support networks lies in their ability to transform what can feel like a solitary struggle into a shared endeavor. They remind you that you're not alone, offering both inspiration and accountability. As you engage with others, you build a community that supports and uplifts you. This sense of belonging can be a powerful motivator, helping you stay committed to your health goals, even when the road gets rocky. So, whether you find your tribe online or in person, know that these connections are not just about accountability; they're about building a life filled with support, understanding, and shared joy.

As we wrap up this chapter on building a support network for accountability, it's clear that having a group or partner to lean on can enhance motivation and commitment. These connections, whether virtual or in-person, create a strong foundation for achieving health goals. With this support, you're better equipped to face challenges and celebrate successes. Moving forward, we'll explore how to integrate these tools and resources into a holistic approach to well-being, ensuring that you have the support you need to thrive.

SO... SHOULD I INTERMITTENT FAST OR NOT?

It all comes down to this question, doesn't it? There's a growing buzz about fasting—a wellness trend that seems to be everywhere these days. Everywhere you look, someone is talking about how fasting is the ultimate solution for women over 50. Lose weight, balance hormones, extend your life—it sounds like a miracle, right?

But here's the truth that rarely gets spoken: You don't have to fast. Not now, not ever—if your body is already working well.

If you want to try this option, let me remind you what you should be aware of:

FINDING YOUR SWEET SPOT: MAKING FASTING WORK FOR YOU

We've learned that hormonal balance is a key player in this game, particularly as we navigate the ups and downs of menopause. We've also explored the profound connection between our physical health and our emotional well-being.

Let's wrap this all up with some real talk. We've covered a lot of ground together – from keeping your muscles strong to managing your mental health, from protecting your bones to exercising safely. Now it's time to put it all together in a way that makes sense for YOUR life.

THE BIG PICTURE: WHAT WE'VE LEARNED

Fasting Is Personal (Like, Really Personal)

Remember when we talked about how everyone's body is different? That wasn't just nice talk. Your fasting journey is as unique as your fingerprint, and here's why:

- Your hormones have their own rhythm
- Your lifestyle has specific demands
- Your health history tells its own story
- Your goals are uniquely yours

Listen to Your Body (It's Smarter Than Any App)

Throughout all our chapters, one theme kept popping up:

- Some days you'll feel like a fasting superhero
- On other days, you'll need more fuel
- Both are perfectly okay
- Your body knows what it needs

Creating Your Personal Fasting Framework

Step 1: Know Your Non-Negotiables

Think about what matters most to you:

- Your health conditions
- Your energy needs
- Your social life
- Your exercise routine
- Your sleep quality

Step 2: Choose Your Approach

Based on what we've discussed:

- Start with a gentle approach
- Adjust as you learn
- Keep what works
- Drop what doesn't

Step 3: Build Your Support System

Remember to:

- Keep healthcare providers in the loop
- Have friends or family who understand
- Know where to get help if needed
- Stay connected with reliable information

MAKING IT SUSTAINABLE: YOUR LONG-TERM SUCCESS PLAN

The Flexibility Factor

Life isn't static, and your fasting shouldn't be either:

- Seasons change (and so will your needs)
- Special occasions happen
- Work demands fluctuate
- Energy levels vary

Your Success Toolkit

Keep these tools handy:

- Knowledge of your body's signals
- Strategies for different situations
- Backup plans for tough days
- Ways to track what works

Common Pitfalls and How to Avoid Them

The "All or Nothing" Trap

Watch out for:

- Thinking one "break" ruins everything
- Getting too rigid with rules
- Competing with others
- Ignoring your body's signals

The Comparison Game

Remember:

- Your journey is yours alone
- Social media isn't the reality
- Progress isn't linear
- Success looks different for everyone

Special Considerations to Keep in Mind

Life Stages Matter

Your needs change with:

- Hormonal shifts
- Age-related changes
- Life transitions
- Health developments

Lifestyle Factors

Consider how fasting fits with the following:

- Your work schedule
- Family responsibilities
- Social commitments
- Exercise routine
- Sleep patterns

Your Personal Fasting Success Checklist

Daily Check-ins:

✓ Energy levels ✓ Mood and mental state ✓ Physical feelings ✓ Sleep quality ✓ Stress levels

Weekly Reviews:

✓ Overall wellbeing ✓ Exercise performance ✓ Social interactions ✓ Emotional health ✓ Progress toward goals

Monthly Assessments:

✓ Health markers ✓ Lifestyle fit ✓ Need for adjustments ✓ Long-term sustainability ✓ Overall satisfaction

When to Celebrate Success

Remember, success isn't just about numbers. Celebrate when:

- You better understand your body
- You make choices that honor your needs
- You maintain balance in your life
- You feel energized and well
- You find your sustainable rhythm

When to Press Pause

It's okay to step back when:

- Your health needs attention
- Life gets overwhelming
- Your body needs more support
- Your mental health requires care

- Something just feels off

Moving Forward: Your Action Plan

1. **Start Where You Are**
    - Assess your current situation
    - Set realistic expectations
    - Begin gradually
    - Build consistently
2. **Stay Flexible**
    - Adapt to life changes
    - Modify as needed
    - Learn from experience
    - Grow with knowledge
3. **Keep Learning**
    - Stay informed about your health
    - Learn from your experiences
    - Connect with reliable resources
    - Share with others when comfortable

The Bottom Line: Your Fasting, Your Way

Remember these final thoughts:

Your Body, Your Rules

- There's no one "right" way to fast
- Your needs may change over time
- What works for others might not work for you
- That's absolutely okay

Success Is Personal

- Define it for yourself
- Celebrate small wins
- Learn from challenges
- Keep growing and adjusting

Health Comes First

- Physical well-being matters
- Mental health is crucial
- Balance is essential
- Sustainability is key

WHEN FASTING IS UNNECESSARY

Listen to your body: If your energy is stable, your blood work looks good, and you feel strong, why would you want to mess with something that's already working perfectly? Fasting isn't a mandatory passport to good health—it's just one potential tool, and not everyone needs it.

The messages bombarding women in midlife can be relentless:

- "You must control your diet."
- "This is how you stay young."
- "You're falling behind if you're not fasting."

But these are just noise.

The Real Cost of Unnecessary Fasting

For women navigating the changes of midlife, adding fasting can create more problems than solutions. Your body is already experiencing significant shifts:

- Hormonal changes
- Metabolic adjustments
- Muscle mass fluctuations

Forcing an additional stress like fasting can lead to:

- Unexpected fatigue
- Irritability
- Disrupted sleep
- Potential muscle loss

Your body has spent decades developing a delicate balance. It knows how to function best with a consistent nutrient supply. Unless a medical professional identifies a specific reason, there's no inherent advantage to restricting your eating.

Breaking Free from Trend Pressure

It's incredibly easy to fall into the trap of thinking you "should" do something just because everyone else is doing it. But health isn't a one-size-fits-all equation. If you're already:

- Maintaining a stable weight
- Feeling energetic
- Experiencing good digestion
- Feeling generally healthy

Then, you have zero obligation to change your approach.

The Power of Trusting Your Current Approach

Many women over 50 thrive on a consistent, balanced approach to eating. Nourishing meals at regular intervals can be exactly what your body needs. No complicated schedules. No restrictive windows. Just good, wholesome nutrition that supports your body's natural rhythms.

THANK YOU FOR JOINING ME ON THIS JOURNEY

Women's solidarity counts!

"The more you give, the more you get back."

— *UNKNOWN*

As you close this book, I want to take a moment to express my heartfelt gratitude for taking the time to explore the insights shared here. If you're a woman over 50, navigating the changes in your body and wondering if intermittent fasting is right for you, I hope this book has provided clarity, support, and guidance to help you make the best choices for your health and well-being.

The journey to understanding our bodies and how to nourish them properly during this time of life is not always easy, but it is incredibly rewarding. And now that you've learned how intermittent fasting might or might not fit into your routine, I invite you to share your experience with others.

Reviews are a powerful way to help spread knowledge and support others who might be on the same path. Your feedback could be the key to helping another woman find the answers she's been searching for. It takes just a moment, and it could change someone's life for the better.

By leaving a review, you could help:

- One more woman find the confidence to take control of her health
- One more woman discover a balanced approach to fasting and weight loss
- One more woman feel understood and empowered during this phase of life
- One more woman make informed decisions that will improve her energy and well-being

If you feel inspired to leave a review, simply scan the QR code below and share your thoughts:

Wishing you health, balance, and joy on your journey,

Eden Thayer

YOUR FINAL TAKEAWAY

Fasting isn't about perfection – it's about finding what works for you in a way that enhances your life rather than restricting it. Whether you fast occasionally, regularly, or decide it's not for you right now, what matters most is that you're making informed choices that support your overall well-being.

Remember, you're not just following a fasting plan; you're creating a sustainable lifestyle that works for YOU. Trust yourself, honor your body's wisdom, and keep moving forward in a way that feels right for your unique journey.

Be kind to yourself along the way. Your body is doing its best every single day, and so are you.

You do not have to fast. You do not need to experiment. You do not need to wonder if you're missing out.

If your health is good, fasting is simply unnecessary.

Trust the habits that have already been serving you well. Your body, with its decades of wisdom, knows exactly what it needs. Sometimes, the most revolutionary act is simply listening to it.

Trust me, I know….

Eden Thayer

REFERENCES

AARP. (n.d.). *Is intermittent fasting safe for people over 50?* Retrieved from https://www.aarp.org/health/healthy-living/info-2024/is-intermittent-fasting-safe-for-older-adults.html

Bodyspec. (n.d.). *Intermittent fasting by age chart: A comprehensive guide.* Retrieved from https://www.bodyspec.com/blog/post/intermittent_fasting_by_age_chart_a_comprehensive_guide

By Winona. (n.d.). *15 foods that help restore hormone balance.* Retrieved from https://bywinona.com/journal/foods-for-hormone-balance?srsltid=AfmBOorE6dQzHPzqonqLb-RDDPAb3PBkseQvc15OIUMGWKG4KACXtSno

By Winona. (n.d.). *Intermittent fasting and menopause: Tips & benefits.* Retrieved from https://bywinona.com/journal/intermittent-fasting-and-menopause?srsltid=AfmBOoqAn19ZrUKebs1hcDd62oB9ixYlQzPnJA54ygLSaFNS73EKAqAI

Cleveland Clinic. (n.d.). *Is intermittent fasting healthy for women?* Retrieved from https://health.clevelandclinic.org/intermittent-fasting-for-women

Everyday Health. (n.d.). *What midlife women should know about intermittent fasting.* Retrieved from https://www.everydayhealth.com/womens-health/what-midlife-women-should-know-about-intermittent-fasting/

Harvard Nutrition Source. (n.d.). *Mindful eating.* Retrieved from https://nutritionsource.hsph.harvard.edu/mindful-eating/

Healthline. (n.d.). *15 non-scale victories to celebrate for weight loss.* Retrieved from https://www.healthline.com/health/non-scale-victories

Healthline. (n.d.). *Intermittent fasting, high-intensity exercise combo.* Retrieved from https://www.healthline.com/health-news/time-restricted-eating-and-high-intensity-exercise-weight-loss

Healthline. (n.d.). *The 20 best ways to lose weight after 50.* Retrieved from https://www.healthline.com/nutrition/how-to-lose-weight-after-50

Kettering Health. (n.d.). *How strength training can help you post-menopause.* Retrieved from https://ketteringhealth.org/how-strength-training-can-help-you-post-menopause/

Kroma Wellness. (n.d.). *Fasting while traveling: 7 helpful tips.* Retrieved from https://kromawellness.com/blogs/news/fasting-while-traveling-tips

Lifesum. (n.d.). *How to navigate social situations while fasting.* Retrieved from https://lifesum.com/nutrition-explained/how-to-navigate-social-situations-while-fasting

Mayo Clinic. (n.d.). *Mindfulness may ease menopausal symptoms.* Retrieved from https://newsnetwork.mayoclinic.org/discussion/mindfulness-may-ease-menopausal-symptoms/

Medical News Today. (n.d.). *Phytoestrogens: Benefits, risks, and food list.* Retrieved from https://www.medicalnewstoday.com/articles/320630

My Menopause Centre. (n.d.). *10 hacks to combat menopausal weight gain.* Retrieved from https://www.mymenopausecentre.com/blog/10-easy-diet-and-lifestyle-changes-to-combat-and-menopausal-and-perimenopausal-weight-gain/

National Institute on Aging. (n.d.). *Sleep problems and menopause: What can I do?* Retrieved from https://www.nia.nih.gov/health/menopause/sleep-problems-and-menopause-what-can-i-do

Naatlanta. (2023, October 1). *How to choose a health and wellness coach.* Retrieved from https://www.naatlanta.com/2023/10/01/467268/how-to-choose-a-health-and-wellness-coach

PMC. (n.d.). *Effect of time-restricted eating on sex hormone levels.* Retrieved from https://pmc.ncbi.nlm.nih.gov/articles/PMC9877115/

PMC. (n.d.). *Effects of fasting on the physiological and psychological aspects.* Retrieved from https://pmc.ncbi.nlm.nih.gov/articles/PMC10421233/

PMC. (n.d.). *Nutrition in menopausal women: A narrative review.* Retrieved from https://pmc.ncbi.nlm.nih.gov/articles/PMC8308420/

Psychology Today. (2023, December). *The healing power of storytelling.* Retrieved from https://www.psychologytoday.com/us/blog/un-numb/202312/the-healing-power-of-storytelling

Reifkind, T. (2012). *The Swing: Lose the fat and get fit with this revolutionary kettlebell program.* HarperOne.

ScienceDaily. (2022, October 25). *How intermittent fasting affects female hormones.* Retrieved from https://www.sciencedaily.com/releases/2022/10/221025150257.htm

The Spruce Eats. (n.d.). *The 8 best meal-planning apps.* Retrieved from https://www.thespruceeats.com/best-meal-planning-apps-4766812

Printed in Dunstable, United Kingdom